International Symposium
Clonidine in Hypertension
Geneva, 14th–16th June 1984

Low Dose
Oral and Transdermal Therapy
of Hypertension

Edited by

M. A. Weber, J. I. M. Drayer and R. Kolloch

With Contributions by

L. Aarons, R. J. Anderson, M. Anlauf, P. Balansard, A. Baralla, P. Baumgart,
C. Bies, J. C. Boekhorst, F. Bonte, E. L. Bravo, D. D. Brewer, O.-E. Brodde,
H. Chehabi, L. C. Chu, K. Conry, L. Corradi, M. D. Cressman, T. Danays,
M. Devous, C. Diehm, L. Dow, J. I. M. Drayer, A. van den Ende,
D. J. Enscore, B. Falkner, H. Finster, R. Fogari, Y. Frances, M. S. Golub,
H. Groth, G. P. Guthrie, Jr., A. Haratz, K. Hopkins, A. Jain, J. J. Keirns,
G. S. M. Kellaway, A. M. Khalifa, L. M. Kirk, J. Knüsel, R. Kolloch,
L. Kuhnert, W. St. J. LaCorte, D. T. Lowenthal, W. F. Lubbe,
T. R. MacGregor, H. Maibach, K. M. Matzek, C. Matthews, F. G. McMahon,
R. Michael, H. Mörl, H. M. Müller, A. Overlack, J. Packer, N. Pateisky,
M. A. Pohl, R. S. Porter, H. Pozenel, W. G. Reed, M. Rowland, J. R. Ryan,
M. P. Sambhi, P. Sans, S. D. Saris, M. Searle, J. E. Shaw, E. Stokeley,
K. O. Stumpe, C. Thananopavarn, R. G. L. van Tol, H. A. Trauth,
H. Vetter, W. Vetter, R. G. A. van Wayjen, M. A. Weber

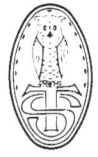

Springer-Verlag Berlin Heidelberg GmbH

Michael A. Weber, M.D.
Jan I. M. Drayer, M.D.
Hypertension Center
Veterans Administration Medical Center
5901 East Seventh Street
Long Beach, CA 90822
U.S.A.

Dr. R. Kolloch
Medizinische Universitäts-Poliklinik
Wilhelmstraße 35–37
5300 Bonn 1
F.R.G.

CIP-Kurztitelaufnahme der Deutschen Bibliothek
Low dose oral and transdermal therapy of hypertension / [Internat. Symposium Clonidine in Hyper-
tension, Geneva, 14–16 June 1984]. Ed. by M. A. Weber . . . With contributions by L. Aarons . . . –
Darmstadt: Steinkopff, 1985.
ISBN 978-3-642-53787-5   ISBN 978-3-642-53785-1 (eBook)
DOI 10.1007/978-3-642-53785-1

NE: Weber, Michael A. [Hrsg.]; Aarons, L. [Mitverf.]; International Symposium Clonidine in Hypertension < 1984, Genève >

Editorial Assistance: Juliane K. Weller – Copy Editing: Cynthia Feast – Production: Heinz J. Schäfer

Contents

Introduction

This book brings together papers presented at an international symposium on centrally-acting antihypertensive agents held in Geneva, Switzerland, in association with the 10th Scientific Meeting of the International Society of Hypertension. A major focus of this symposium was the sympatholytic agent, clonidine, and was partly stimulated by the recent development of an innovative transdermal system for administering this antihypertensive drug.

Although clonidine has been available to clinicians for several years, there has been a recent reawakening of interest in this type of medication. The centrally-acting antihypertensive agents appear to be effective both as monotherapy and in combination with other drugs. There are no significant contraindications to their use, and they do not appear to produce metabolic side effects. In this symposium we have paid attention to two types of patients: those with uncomplicated mild hypertension, and those with more difficult forms of hypertension associated with concurrent conditions.

Mild hypertension is very common and poses some interesting problems. There is evidence that antihypertensive treatment decreases death rate and the incidence of hypertensive cardiovascular complications in these patients, but there is concern that treatment can of itself cause difficulties for some individuals. Systemic and central nervous system side effects have been observed with virtually all antihypertensive agents, including placebo, and potentially may have a negative impact on the quality of life of patients who otherwise have an asymptomatic condition. Moreover, certain agents have the potential for inducing unwanted metabolic effects, including changes in plasma concentrations of electrolytes, lipids, and glucose. It may be partly for these reasons that the benefits of long-term therapy for mild hypertension have sometimes been less than anticipated.

It can be useful to consider antihypertensive therapy on the basis of special categories of patients. For example, age and other demographic factors might have an influence on treatment responsiveness. Conditions such as renal insufficiency or diabetes mellitus that often coexist with hypertension can also influence the choice of treatment. This book addresses several of these issues. Specifically, we have examined characteristics of the sympatholytic agent, clonidine, and the ways in which it can contribute to the management of various forms of hypertension.

New delivery systems for pharmacological agents always arouse interest, but the development of a transdermal therapeutic system for clonidine has evoked particularly close attention. This book contains results of some of the preliminary studies with this new treatment system. The early data indicate that the transdermal clonidine is as efficacious as the oral form of the drug, and appears to have the virtue of producing only minimal systemic side effects.

As is appropriate for investigators evaluating a new approach to treatment, we have looked closely at any special problems that might be related to this method of administration. For example, there is discussion in this book concerning the dermatological consequences of applying a therapeutic system directly to the skin for seven-day treatment periods. There have been some reports of local skin reactions under the areas where the transdermal systems have been placed, although these tend to be mild and to disappear rapidly when treatment is discontinued. It is of interest, too, that there appears to be a difference in the incidence of this type of reaction between investigators in different geographical areas. Of importance, there have been no reports of generalized allergic responses or of systemic manifestations during treatment with the transdermal system. The developmental work with this method of treatment is still continuing, but it is expected that this innovative system will be available for clinical use in the near future.

The chief emphasis of this book has been on the importance of low-dose antihypertensive therapy. Indeed, the transdermal clonidine system, which is both efficacious and well tolerated, provides doses of drug which are lower than those usually administered with oral therapy. This information, together with growing data from studies employing very low doses of oral clonidine, points out a potentially new direction for the use of this well-established agent. We hope that the reader will find this book to be of practical as well as of theoretical interest, and that perhaps it might help point the way to rewarding new approaches for managing the large numbers of patients with milder forms of hypertension.

Long Beach, California, and Bonn, F.R.G.

Michael A. Weber
Jan I. M. Drayer
Rainer E. Kolloch

Cardiovascular and Neurohumoral Effects of Long-Term Oral Clonidine Monotherapy in Essential Hypertensive Patients

Emmanuel L. Bravo, Michael D. Cressman, and Marc A. Pohl

Introduction

The hypothesis of a neurogenic component in essential hypertension has had a long and controversial history; increased sympathetic nervous activity may play a significant role in both the initiation and maintenance of hypertension. However, in human hypertension the investigation of the sympathetic nervous system is complicated by the need to rely on indirect means of investigation. The main lines of evidence have consisted of the haemodynamic pattern in early hypertension, the increased vascular responsiveness to exogenous catecholamines, and the hypotensive effect of sympatholytic drugs. In the present study we sought to obtain more direct evidence by correlating plasma noradrenaline levels with arterial pressure levels before and after interruption of the sympathetic nervous system with clonidine, a centrally-acting sympathetic inhibitor.

Methods

Eighteen patients with untreated essential hypertension were studied. All studies were conducted in the outpatient department; patients were told to remain on their usual diets and not to vary them during the course of the studies, which lasted for seven weeks. In the first week control measurements were obtained, followed by four weeks of treatment, then two weeks without treatment. On the seventh day of each weekly period, patients were asked to collect a 24-hour urine specimen for measurement of excretion rates of sodium, potassium and aldosterone. They then fasted overnight and reported to the outpatient department at 0800 hours. Patients were weighed, then a 19-gauge scalp vein needle was inserted into an antecubital vein and kept patent with heparinized saline. After 30 minutes of supine rest, blood pressure (BP) and heart rate (HR) were measured three times, five minutes apart. Then blood for the measurement of plasma catecholamines and plasma renin activity (PRA) was obtained. In some patients, blood volume measurements

Research Division, Cleveland Clinic Foundation, Cleveland, Ohio, U.S.A.

were also made. BP, HR and plasma catecholamines were again obtained after five minutes' quiet standing. After the first visit, patients started with clonidine 0.1 mg twice daily. If during the weekly visits supine diastolic BP exceeded 90 mmHg, clonidine was increased by 0.2 mg increments per week up to a maximum dose of 0.6 mg per day during the four-week treatment period. During the recovery period, the drug dose was reduced slowly over a three-day period.

Brachial arterial pressure was measured indirectly with a mercury sphygmomanometer; HR was determined from the radial pulse. Plasma catecholamines, PRA, and blood volume were measured by previously described procedures (Bravo et al. 1975 and Bravo et al. 1981). Results were expressed as group averages ± SEM. Spearman correlation coefficients were used to analyze the relationship between the neurohumoral and cardiovascular responses.

Results

Before treatment, systolic BP (SBP), diastolic BP (DBP), HR and plasma NA averaged 158 ± 6 mmHg, 104 ± 2 mmHg, 74 ± 3 beats/min, and 239 ± 25 pg/ml, respectively (Fig. 1). With treatment, BP, HR, and plasma NA were all reduced significantly after the first week and remained so during the entire four-week treatment period. After discontinuation of clonidine, BP, HR, and plasma NA all returned to near pretreatment values. There were no associated changes in either blood volume, body weight, or PRA, which suggests that the fall in BP with clonidine was mostly as a result of inhibition of the sympathetic nervous system.

Fig. 1. Effect of clonidine monotherapy on supine blood pressure, heart rate and plasma noradrenaline (Mean ± SEM). * Significantly different from control.

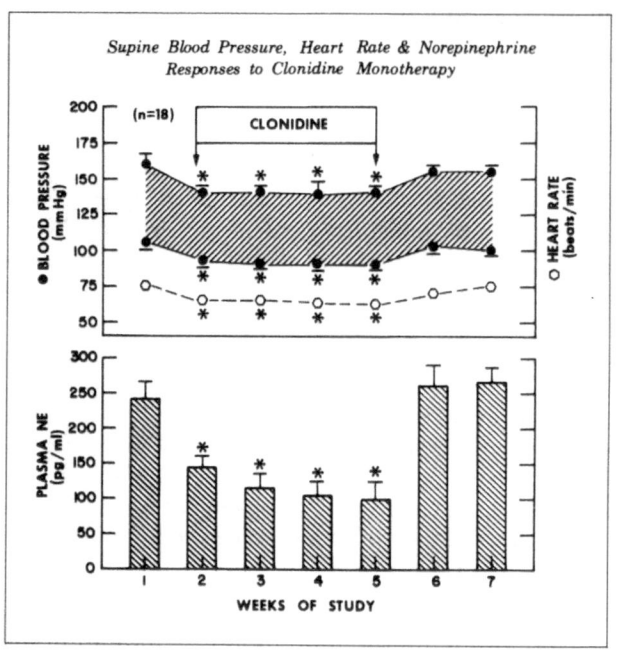

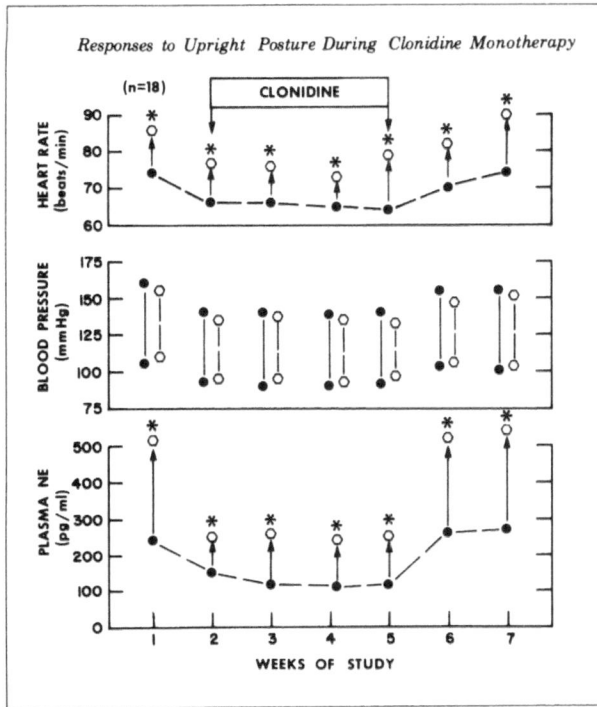

Fig. 2. Effect of upright posture on heart rate, blood pressure, and plasma noradrenaline during clonidine monotherapy. * Significantly different from supine resting values.

Before treatment, significant correlations were found between basal plasma NA and HR ($r = 0.64$, $p < 0.05$), SBP ($r = 0.57$, $p < 0.05$) and DBP ($r = 0.54$, $p < 0.05$); patients with the highest basal plasma NA levels had the highest HRs and BPs. With treatment, the levels of basal plasma NA correlated significantly with the percentage fall in both SBP ($r = 0.75$, $p < 0.01$) and DBP ($r = 0.72$, $p < 0.01$). Further, the percentage fall in plasma NA also correlated with the percentage reduction of SBP ($r = 0.52$, $p < 0.05$) and DBP ($r = 0.71$, $p < 0.01$).

Before treatment, there were quick and significant increases in HR and plasma NA; since SBP fell and DBP increased, there was essentially no change in mean arterial pressure. During treatment, the cardiovascular and neurohumoral responses to upright posture were preserved, which prevented the occurrence of orthostatic hypotension.

Discussion

In this study, we have found further evidence for a role of sympathetic mechanisms in the maintenance of high blood pressure in some patients with essential hypertension. We found that patients with the highest plasma NA levels not only had the highest heart rates and blood pressures, but also had the greatest reductions in blood pressure during long-term sympathetic inhibition with clonidine. A possible causal relationship between sympathetic nerve activity and blood pressure regulation is supported by the fact that reductions in blood pressure were directly related to decreases in plasma NA, a measure of car-

5

diovascular sympathetic nervous system activity (Goldstein et al. 1983). Failure to demonstrate associated changes in blood volume, body weight, and plasma renin activity agrees with the results from other studies (Sambhi 1983). These findings are consistent with the concept that the antihypertensive effect of clonidine is mainly related to its ability to inhibit central sympathetic outflow, resulting in decreased NA release (and thus in circulating plasma NA) (Kobinger 1978).

The effects of clonidine on blood pressure can be explained by its known haemodynamic actions. Sambhi et al. (1983) found that clonidine given over a three-month period consistently reduced heart rate and total peripheral resistance without any change in cardiac output. Because heart rate was significantly reduced and cardiac output remained unchanged, stroke volume increased slightly but significantly. By contrast, Lund-Johansen observed that after one year of different doses of clonidine, there was a slight decline in cardiac output and no significant change in the calculated peripheral resistance (Lund-Johansen 1974). These contrasting results may be attributable to differences in experimental design and doses of the drug.

Clonidine effectively decreased supine resting plasma NA; however, it did not inhibit plasma NA increases induced by upright posture. This finding agrees with previous observations that clonidine is more potent in reducing spontaneous discharges than in suppressing induced discharges in the sympathetic nervous system (Kobinger 1978). This could also account for the absence of orthostatic hypotension during these studies.

In summary, clonidine monotherapy reduced systolic and diastolic blood pressure; this was associated with significant and consistent decreases in heart rate and plasma NA with preservation of the cardiovascular and neurohumoral responses to upright posture. Patients with the highest pretreatment plasma NA values had the greatest reductions in blood pressure with clonidine. This suggests that enhanced sympathetic activity contributes to maintenance of raised blood pressure in some patients with essential hypertension. Furthermore, combining plasma NA measurements with pharmacological interruption of the sympathetic nervous system may be a reasonable approach by which to assess the neurogenic component of some hypertensive states.

Acknowledgement

The authors would like to thank Boehringer Ingelheim Ltd. for the generous gift of clonidine that was used in these studies.

References

1. Bravo EL, Tarazi RC, Dustan HP (1975) Beta-adrenergic blockade in diuretic-treated essential hypertension. N Engl J Med 292: 66–70
2. Bravo EL, Tarazi RC, Fouad FM, Vidt DG, Gifford RW Jr (1981) Clonidine suppression test: a useful aid in the diagnosis of pheochromocytoma. N Engl J Med 305: 623–626
3. Goldstein DS, McCarty R, Polinsky RJ, Kopin IJ (1983) Relationship between plasma norepinephrine and sympathetic neural activity. Hypertension 5: 552–559
4. Kobinger W (1978) Central alpha-adrenergic systems as targets for hypotensive drugs. Rev. Physiol Biochem Pharmacol 81: 40–100
5. Lund-Johansen P (1974) Hemodynamic changes at rest and during exercise in long-term clonidine therapy of essential hypertension. Acta Med Scand 195: 111–115

6. Sambhı MP (1983) Clonidine monotherapy in mild and moderate hypertension. In: Hayduk K, Bock KD (eds) Central Blood Pressure Regulation: The Role of α_2-Receptor Stimulation. Steinkopff Verlag, Darmstadt

Authors' address:
Emmanuel L. Bravo, M.D.
Research Division
Cleveland Clinic Foundation
9500 Euclid Avenue
Cleveland, Ohio 44106
U.S.A.

Alpha-Adrenoceptor Density and Clonidine

Otto-Erich Brodde, Adel M. Khalifa, and Manfred Anlauf

Alpha-adrenoceptors are involved in blood pressure regulation at different sites of the central nervous system and at the peripheral sympathetic vascular junctions (Kobinger 1978). The region of the nucleus tractus solitarii especially shows a high density of α-adrenoceptors, mainly of the α_2-subtype. This nucleus processes information from higher parts of the brain and from the baroreceptors. Stimulation of these α_2-adrenoceptors reduces the peripheral sympathetic tone and enhances the vagal tone (Fig. 1). Consequently blood pressure and heart rate are lowered. The α-adrenoceptors at the peripheral sympathetic vascular junctions may play different roles: at postsynaptic sites α_1- and α_2-adrenoceptors are involved in the constriction of resistance vessels (Timmermans and Van Zwieten 1981), whereas presynaptic α_2-receptors are assumed to modulate noradrenaline release by a negative feedback mechanism. Stimulation of these presynaptic α_2-adrenoceptors by endogenous noradrenaline or exogenously applied agonists depresses the sympathetic activity (Starke 1977).

In the past ten years it has become possible to investigate adrenergic receptors on the molecular level by means of radioligand binding studies (Hoffman and Lefkowitz 1980). While in animals the organs are directly accessible, in human beings circulating blood cells have been proved to be a suitable tool to study α- and β-adrenoceptor alterations (Motulsky and Insel 1982).

Platelets containing a homogeneous population of α_2-adrenoceptors, which mediate aggregation (Grant and Scrutton 1979) and inhibit adenylate cyclase activity (Jakobs et al. 1976) are a frequently used model for studies of α-adrenoceptor alterations under various conditions. As radioligand for α_2-adrenoceptors we use ^{3}H-yohimbine (Brodde et al. 1982). Specific binding of ^{3}H-yohimbine to platelet membranes (Fig. 2) is calculated from the difference between total binding and unspecific binding, i.e. binding in the presence of a high concentration of phentolamine (10 μM). The straight line in the Scatchard (1949) plot (inset of Fig. 2) shows that we identify only one population of adrenoceptors.

In our experiments we tried to answer the following questions:

Firstly: Do differences exist in α_2-adrenoceptor density between normotensive and hypertensive subjects?

Secondly: Does an in vitro and in vivo stimulation of α_2-receptors by clonidine alter density and function of receptors?

Biochemical Research Laboratory, Medizinische Klinik & Poliklinik, Division of Rena & Hypertensive Diseases, University of Essen, F.R.G.

8

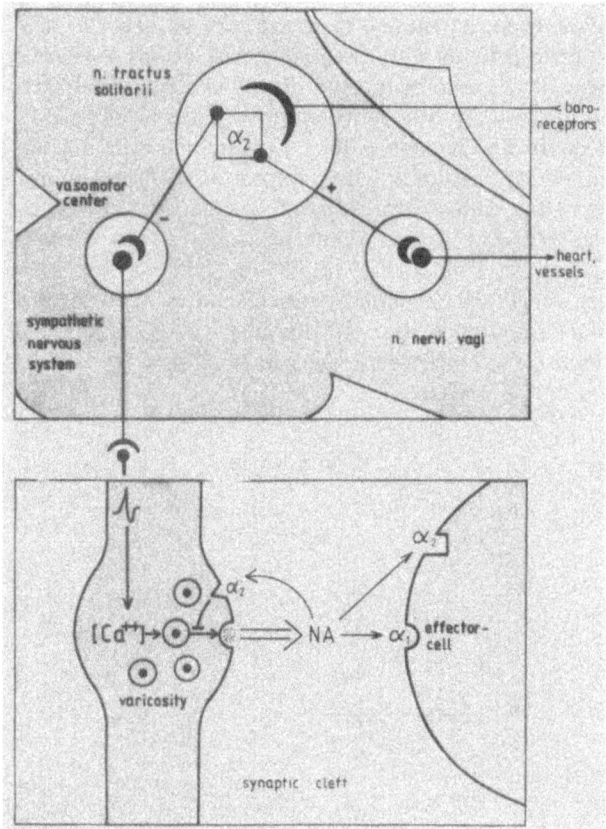

Fig. 1. Regulation of noradrenaline release by central and peripheral mechanisms. In the central nervous system (nucleus tractus solitarii) stimulation of α_2-adrenoceptors decreases sympathetic outflow (–) and increases vagal tone (+). In the periphery (synaptic cleft) stimulation of presynaptic α_2-adrenoceptors inhibits noradrenaline release.

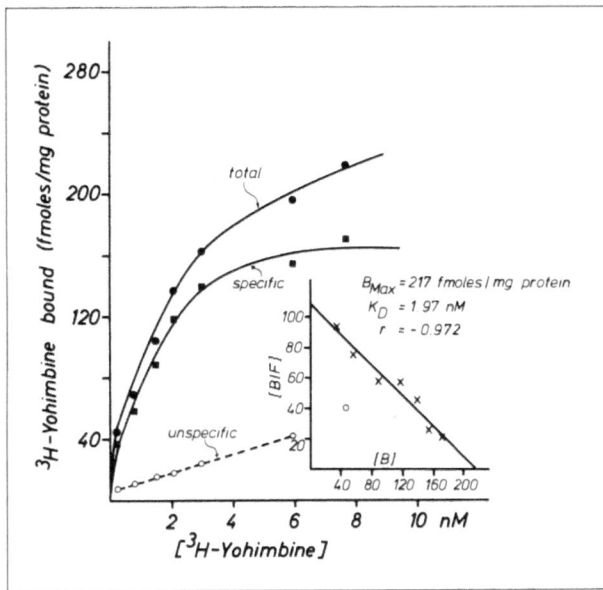

Fig. 2. Binding of ^{3}H-yohimbine to human platelet membranes as function of increasing ^{3}H-yohimbine concentrations. Binding was carried out with various concentrations of ^{3}H-yohimbine ranging from 0.5–10 nM in the absence (●—● = total) and presence (○ - - - ○ = unspecific) of 10 μM phentolamine to determine specific binding (■—■).
Ordinate: ^{3}H-yohimbine bound (fmoles/mg protein).
Abscissa: Free ^{3}H-yohimbine concentration (nM).
Inset: Scatchard-plot (1949) of specific ^{3}H-yohimbine binding. The ratio B/F of specifically bound ^{3}H-yohimbine (fmoles/mg protein) to free ^{3}H-yohimbine (nM) is plotted as function of B = specifically bound ^{3}H-yohimbine.

The concentration of α_2-receptors has been determined in platelets of 40 healthy male normotensives and 40 age-matched male patients with essential hypertension. As can be seen from Fig. 3 the platelets of the control group bound specifically about 170 fmol ^{3}H-yohimbine/mg protein. The density of α_2-receptors in hypertensive patients was significantly higher with 330 fmol/mg protein. The K_D-values for ^{3}H-yohimbine were not significantly different, indicating that the affinity of α_2-adrenoceptors for ^{3}H-yohimbine was not changed. Further analysis of the data gave a negative correlation between α-receptor density and age in normotensives, but suggests a tendency for a positive correlation in hypertensive subjects.

Considering the correlation between mean arterial blood pressure and α_2-adrenoceptor density resulted in a highly significant positive correlation with an r-value of 0.591 and an unbroken transition from normotensive to hypertensive subjects (Fig. 4).

Fig. 3. α_2-adrenoceptor density in platelets of 40 male healthy volunteers (aged 19–81 years) and 40 male patients with essential hypertension (aged 20–72 years).
Ordinates: α_2-adrenoceptor density (fmoles ^{3}H-yohimbine specifically bound/mg protein).
Solid horizontal lines and broken lines: mean ± S.E.M. of α_2-adrenoceptor density in the respective collective.

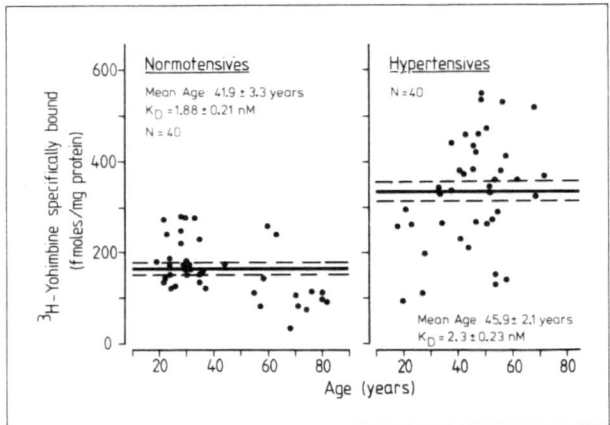

Fig. 4. Correlation between mean arterial blood pressure and α_2-adrenoceptor density in platelets of normotensive (O) and essential hypertensive subjects (●).
Ordinate: α_2-adrenoceptor density (fmoles ^{3}H-yohimbine specifically bound/mg protein).
Abscissa: Mean arterial blood pressure (mmHg).

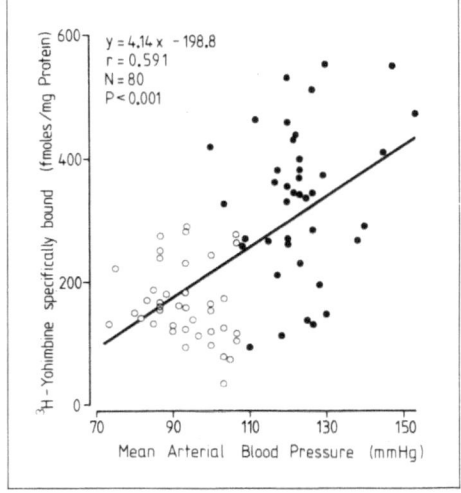

In vivo and in vitro studies have shown that the adrenoceptor number rather than being a static entity is dynamically regulated by a variety of drugs, hormones, and (patho)physiological conditions. Chronic stimulation by an agonist leads to a reduction in receptor density ("down-regulation") and vice versa chronic inhibition by antagonists (without ISA) to an increase in receptor density ("up-regulation") (Lefkowitz 1982).

Incubation of human platelet membranes with various concentrations of clonidine for 16 hours at 25 °C led to a decrease of the maximal number of binding sites (Fig. 5). The reductions of B_{max} amounted to 9.2, 18.3 and 26.4% when the concentration of clonidine was increased from $10^{-6}-10^{-4}$ M, whereas the α-adrenoceptor antagonist phentolamine did not affect the B_{max}-values. The affinity of ^{3}H-yohimbine to α_2-adrenoceptors, however, was not changed, as indicated by the nearly identical K_D-values.

The desensitization of α_2-receptors can also be demonstrated in a different way. Binding of agonists to α_2-adrenoceptors can be modulated by guanyl nucleotides (Michel et al. 1980). In vitro, in not incubated platelet membranes clonidine inhibits ^{3}H-yohimbine binding with a shallow displacement curve (Fig. 6) indicating heterogeneous binding to

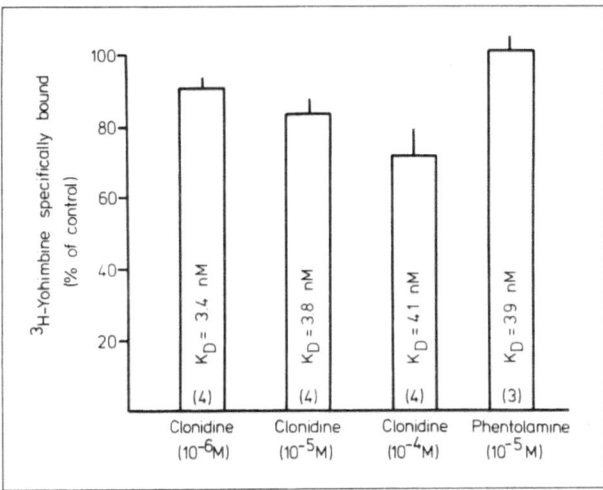

Fig. 5. Influence of preincubation with clonidine ($10^{-6}-10^{-4}$ M) or phentolamine (10^{-5} M) on ^{3}H-yohimbine binding to human platelet membranes.

Ordinate: Maximal number of ^{3}H-yohimbine binding sites (determined by Scatchard-analysis) in per cent of control (i.e. in membranes preincubated with 50 mM Tris 0.5 mM EDTA buffer pH 7.5 = 100%; B_{max} amounted in these membranes to 199.7 ± 17.3 fmoles bound/mg protein, n = 8). Means ± S.E.M.; number of experiments at the bottom of each column.

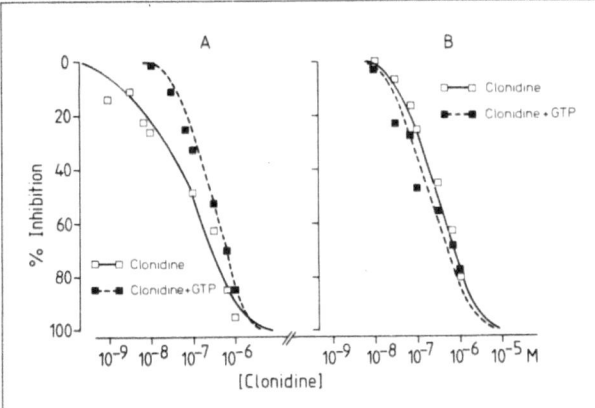

Fig. 6. Influence of GTP (10^{-4} M) on inhibition of specific ^{3}H-yohimbine binding (5 nM) to control (A) and desensitized (B) human platelet membranes by clonidine.

Ordinate: Inhibition of binding in per cent (inhibition by 10 μM phentolamine = 100%).

Abscissa: Molar concentration of clonidine. Each value is the mean of 4 experiments with a S.E.M. < 4%.

two affinity states of the α_2-adrenoceptor. In the presence of GTP (10^{-4} M) the curve is shifted to the right and steepened. But if the same procedure is repeated in platelet membranes preincubated with clonidine (Fig. 6B) identical steep inhibition curves are found, independent of whether GTP was present or not.

These results indicate that "down-regulation" of α_2-adrenoceptors by clonidine impairs binding of agonists to the high affinity state of the receptor.

The desensitization of platelet α_2-adrenoceptors by clonidine can be also demonstrated by in vivo experiments. This is demonstrated in Fig. 7, which shows the influence of an oral clonidine treatment (150 μg, 3 times daily for a week) on the number of platelet α_2-adrenoceptors, plasma catecholamine concentration, blood pressure and heart rate in 3 hypertensive patients, 1 male, 2 females. Blood pressure was reduced from 155/107 mmHg to 125/80 mmHg and heart rate from 90 to 72 beats/min. Plasma catecholamines and ^{3}H-yohimbine binding sites were significantly reduced after three days of clonidine treatment and remained at reduced levels throughout the period of treatment. After withdrawal of clonidine, blood pressure, heart rate, and plasma catecholamines rapidly increased and after two days had reached values similar to or higher than before treatment. ^{3}H-yohimbine binding sites, however, continued to decrease for about two days after cessation of clonidine, before they returned to control values within a further two days.

In a further series of experiments α_2-receptor sensitivity in platelets taken from control subjects and clonidine-treated patients was assessed by inhibition of ^{3}H-yohimbine binding with clonidine (Fig. 8B) and with adrenaline (Fig. 8A). As in the in vitro experiments with clonidine incubation, clonidine treatment resulted in steep monophasic curves in contrast to the shallow curves of untreated controls. Addition of GTP (10^{-4} M)

Fig. 7. Influence of clonidine treatment (3×150 μg/d for 7 days) on the number of α_2-adrenoceptors in platelet membranes, plasma catecholamine concentration, blood pressure and heart rate in hypertensive patients.
Ordinate, Upper Panel: Maximal number of ^{3}H-yohimbine binding sites (determined by Scatchard-analysis ●—●) in per cent of control (i.e. value before treatment: ^{3}H-yohimbine bound 158.1 ± 11.2 fmoles/mg protein, n = 3, left); plasma catecholamine concentration (adrenaline + noradrenaline O—O) in per cent of control (i.e. value before treatment = 0.55 ± 0.11 ng/ml, n = 3, right). Lower Panel: blood pressure in mmHg and heart rate in beats/min. Means $\pm$ S.E.M. of 3 experiments performed on three patients.

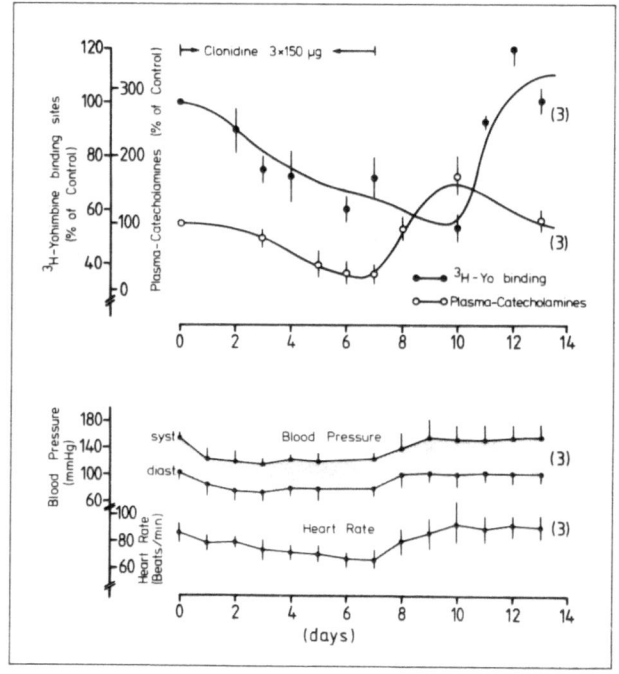

12

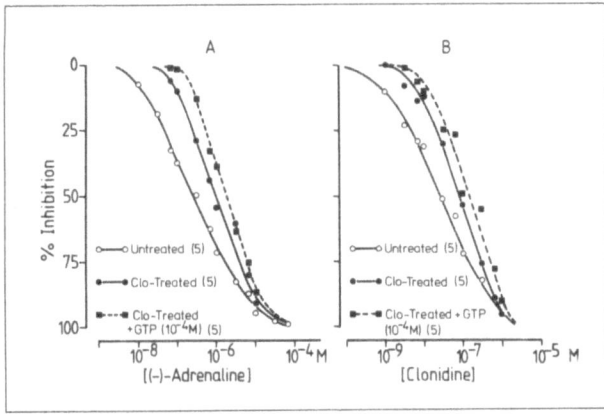

Fig. 8. Inhibition of specific ^{3}H-yohimbine binding (5 nM) in platelet membranes derived from hypertensive patients treated with clonidine (3×150 μg/d and 3×300 μg/d for at least three weeks) or from untreated controls by (–)-adrenaline (A) and clonidine (B). Ordinate: Inhibition of binding in per cent (inhibition by 10 μM phentolamine = 100%).
Abscissa: Molar concentrations of adrenaline or clonidine. Means of 5 experiments performed on 5 subjects in each group with a S.E.M. < 3%.

○—○ Membranes from untreated subjects; ●—● Membranes from clonidine-treated subjects ■----■ Membranes from clonidine-treated subjects after addition of GTP (10^{-4} M) to the incubation mixture.

could not further displace significantly the curves of clonidine treated patients. Nearly identical results were observed when the physiological agonist adrenaline instead of clonidine (Fig. 8A) was used.

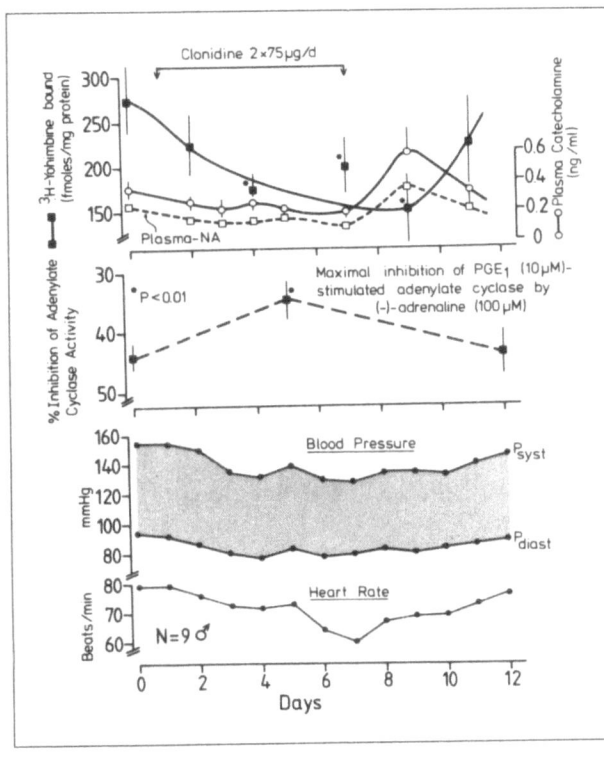

Fig. 9. Influence of clonidine (2×75 μg/d for 7 days) on the number of α_2-adrenoceptors in platelets, plasma catecholamines, (–)-adrenaline-induced inhibition of PGE$_1$-stimulated platelet adenylate cyclase, blood pressure, and heart rate in 9 male hypertensive patients.
Ordinates (left) from top to bottom: Platelet α_2-adrenoceptor number in fmoles ^{3}H-yohimbine bound/mg protein (■—■); maximal inhibition of PGE$_1$-stimulated adenylate cyclase activity by (–)-adrenaline in per cent; blood pressure in mmHg and heart rate in beats/min. Right: plasma catecholamines (○—○) and plasma noradrenaline (□----□) in ng/ml. Means ± S.E.M. of 9 experiments performed in 9 patients.

13

Because of the small number of patients and because of probable sex differences, our first experiences with clonidine treatment and its influence on α-receptor density are open to scepticism. Therefore we repeated the experiments in nine male hypertensive patients (Fig. 9) also treated for one week, but only with 75 μg clonidine twice a day. Treatment resulted in a decrease of blood pressure and heart rate. The reduction of α_2-binding sites and its time course were nearly identical to the first experiment. Immediately after cessation of treatment catecholamine levels exceeded the pretreatment values whereas the depression of receptors outlasted the treatment for two days.

The middle graph of the figure demonstrates that not only receptor density but also receptor function has been changed under clonidine treatment, since the inhibitory effect of 10^{-4} M adrenaline on PGE_1-stimulated adenylate cyclase activity in platelets was significantly diminished. This is illustrated in more detail in Fig. 10 which shows that after four days of clonidine treatment the concentration-response curve for the inhibitory effect of adrenaline on PGE_1-stimulated adenylate cyclase activity was significantly shifted to the right to higher concentrations. Four days after clonidine withdrawal, however, the adrenaline inhibition curve was superimposable on that obtained before treatment.

Fig. 10. Effects of clonidine treatment (2 × 75 μg/d for 7 days) on inhibition of PGE_1-stimulated platelet adenylate cyclase activity by (−)-adrenaline in 9 male hypertensive patients.
Ordinate: Adenylate cyclase activity in per cent of maximal stimulation evoked by 10 μM PGE_1 = 100%.
Abscissa: Molar concentrations of (−)-adrenaline (Means ± S.E.M.).

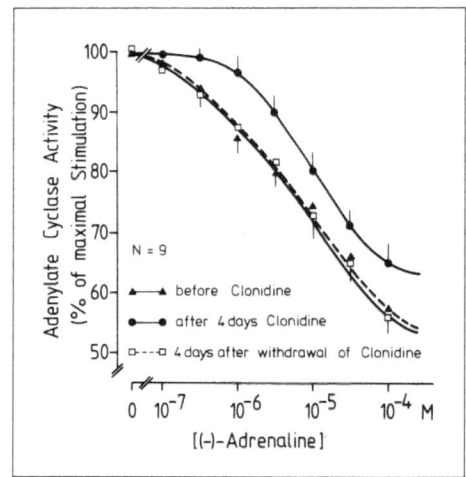

In Summary

1. α-adrenoceptors are involved in blood pressure regulation at different central and peripheral sites of the autonomic nervous system.
2. The density of α_2-adrenoceptors in platelets of primary hypertensive patients is increased when compared with age-matched normotensive subjects.

At present it is difficult to explain the significance of this last finding. α_2-receptors may contribute to an increase or decrease in blood pressure. However, since changes of platelet α_2-adrenoceptors seem to be accompanied by changes of α_1-receptors in the same direction it can be speculated that α_1-receptor density is also enhanced and may therefore contribute to a blood pressure increase in essential hypertension.

3. A short-term oral treatment of mild hypertensives with low and medium doses of clonidine reduces the number and responsiveness of α_2-receptors. This effect outlasts the cessation of treatment for one to two days.

This does not necessarily mean a normalization of α-adrenoceptors as under clonidine treatment the situation of the α_1-type adrenoceptors may be quite different. Down-regulation of α_2-adrenoceptors by the stimulatory activity of the drug may be equalized by an up-regulation of α_1-adrenoceptors as a consequence of a deficient release of the natural agonist noradrenaline.

4. Our findings may contribute to an explanation of the pathogenesis of the rebound phenomenon appearing after cessation of clonidine.

If, as assumed, α_2-receptors are involved in a feedback mechanism for noradrenaline release, their outlasting depression may be the reason for the overshoot of this transmitter.

References

1. Brodde O-E, Hardung A, Ebel H, Bock KD (1982) GTP regulates binding of agonists to α_2-adrenergic receptors in human platelets. Arch Int Pharmacodyn Ther 258: 193–207
2. Grant JA, Scrutton MC (1979) Novel α_2-adrenoceptors primarily responsible for inducing human platelet aggregation. Nature 277: 659–661
3. Hoffman BB, Lefkowitz RJ (1980) Radio-Ligand Binding Studies of adrenergic receptors: new insights into molecular and physiological regulation. Annu Rev Pharmacol Toxicol 20: 581–608
4. Jakobs KH, Saur W, Schultz G (1976) Reduction of adenylate cyclase activity in lysates of human platelets by the alpha-adrenergic component of epinephrine. J Cyclic Nucleotide Res 2: 381–392
5. Kobinger W (1978) Central α-adrenergic systems as target for hypotensive drugs. Rev Physiol Biochem Pharmacol 81: 40–100
6. Lefkowitz RJ (1982) Clinical physiology of adrenergic receptor regulation. Am J Physiol 243: E43–E47
7. Michel T, Hoffman BB, Lefkowitz RJ (1980) Differential regulation of the α_2-adrenergic receptor by Na$^+$ and guanine nucleotides. Nature 288: 709–711
8. Motulsky HJ, Insel PA (1982) Adrenergic receptors in man. Direct identification, physiologic regulation, and clinical alterations. N Eng J Med 307: 18–29
9. Scatchard G (1949) The attraction of proteins for small molecules and ions. Ann NY Acad Sci 51: 660–672
10. Starke K (1977) Regulation of noradrenaline release by presynaptic receptor systems. Rev Physiol Biochem Pharmacol 77: 1–124
11. Timmermans PBMWM, van Zwieten PA (1981) The postsynaptic α_2-adrenoceptor. J Auton Pharmacol 1: 171–183

Authors' address:
Priv.-Doz. Dr. O.-E. Brodde
Biochemical Research Laboratory
Medizinische Klinik und Poliklinik
Division of Renal and Hypertensive Diseases
University of Essen
Hufelandstraße 55
4300 Essen
F.R.G.

Transdermal Clonidine in Elderly Patients with Mild Hypertension: Effects on Blood Pressure and Plasma Catecholamines

Michael S. Golub, Chalemphol Thananopavarn, and Mohinder P. Sambhi

Introduction

Oral clonidine has gained increasing acceptance as initial monotherapy for mild to moderate hypertension (Sambhi 1983). We have reported that this therapy does not significantly change fluid volumes, cardiac haemodynamics or renal function (Thananopavarn et al. 1982). Additionally, the potentially disadvantageous changes in lipid chemistry that have been seen with diuretic and β-blocking drugs have not been reported with clonidine. The development of a transdermal preparation of clonidine has some practical and theoretical advantages which could extend the usefulness of clonidine as initial monotherapy in mild to moderate hypertension. The once-weekly administration is a convenience that could enhance compliance. Also, the consistent blood levels achieved should avoid high peak blood concentrations and thereby reduce drug-related side-effects.

In the elderly there are additional reasons why this therapy might prove effective and desirable; these patients are likely to have loss of compliance in the large arteries. Volume contraction with diuretics or reduction in cardiac output with β-blockers may not be well tolerated in this population. The lack of effects of clonidine on fluid volume, cardiac output and lipid and carbohydrate metabolism are marked advantages in this population. Oral clonidine, with or without a diuretic, is effective therapy in the elderly in our experience (Thananopavarn et al. 1983). Although the contribution of the sympathetic nervous system to hypertension in the elderly is not known precisely, it has been shown that plasma noradrenaline levels increase with age (Weidmann et al. 1978). The ability of clonidine to decrease plasma noradrenaline levels is well documented (Thananopavarn et al. 1982). Blood pressure readings in older subjects vary more than in younger patients with hypertension (Drayer et al. 1982). Therefore, smooth action of the prescribed antihypertensive is desirable to avoid accentuation of this variability. The consistent blood levels achieved with the transdermal patch could be a significant advantage.

We have analysed preliminary data from the first ten subjects aged over 60 years who have entered into a protocol to investigate the acceptability and efficacy of transdermal clonidine in the elderly with mild hypertension.

Division of Hypertension, Sepulveda Veterans Medical Center, UCLA-San Fernando Medical Program, UCLA School of Medicine, Sepulveda, California, U.S.A.

Patients and Methods

The subjects were all male patients aged over 60 years (range 61–72 years, mean 65.5) recruited from the hypertension clinic at Sepulveda Veterans Administration Medical Center. Nine patients were white and one was black.

The protocol was approved by the institutional Human Studies Committee. Patients with significant cardiac, renal, hepatic or metabolic diseases were excluded from participation. All subjects who were taking antihypertensive medications were tapered off. The patients were observed for four weeks off medications. Placebo transdermal patches were placed on the upper arm for the last two weekly visits. Patients with sitting diastolic blood pressure in the 90–104 mmHg range were included in the study. An extension of two further weeks of placebo was allowed for those not qualifying initially. Active medication was begun with a single TTS-1 patch (Transdermal Therapeutic System 1, approximately 0.1 mg clonidine/day) placed on the upper arm. The goal for control was a diastolic pressure below 90 with at least a 5 mmHg decrease from control. Patients not achieving this goal were titrated up on the clonidine dose at weekly intervals as follows: TTS-2 (0.2 mg clonidine/day), TTS-3 (0.3 mg clonidine/day), two TTS-2 (0.4 mg clonidine/day) and two TTS-3 (0.6 mg clonidine/day). If a pressure below goal was achieved, the same dose was repeated for an additional week. Those patients remaining below goal blood pressure were then seen at monthly intervals for three visits and were instructed to change the patches weekly, alternating the site from one side to the other. In those patients whose blood pressure did not remain controlled for two consecutive weekly visits the titration was continued. Those failing to reach goal blood pressure at the highest dose were discontinued from the protocol. Several patients have continued in a nine-month extension of the protocol after completing the three-month stable dose phase. Those subjects discontinuing the patches due to side-effects or failure to control blood pressure were rechecked at 3, 7 and 14 days after discontinuation. For those using two patches, one was removed three days before the final discontinuation of the medication.

Blood pressure (mercury sphygmomanometer) and pulse were measured three times in the sitting (five minutes) and standing (two minutes) positions and averaged at each visit. Serum electrolytes, blood count, urinalysis, and electrocardiograms were performed during the placebo, titration and stable dose periods of the study.

Plasma noradrenaline and adrenaline were determined by radioenzymatic assay (Vlachakis and Mendlowitz 1980) on samples obtained at the completion of the placebo, titration and stable dose phases of the study. The blood was obtained through indwelling butterfly needles placed in the antecubital vein at least 30 minutes previously. The patients remained quietly at rest in the supine position throughout this period.

Results

Nine of the 10 subjects achieved goal blood pressure levels. One subject did not show any fall in blood pressure with the highest dose and was discontinued from the protocol. The dosage of clonidine required for desired control is presented in Table 1. The blood pressure measurements in the sitting and standing positions decreased significantly (p < 0.001) in the nine responding patients at the completion of the titration phase and remained significantly decreased (p < 0.001) in the six subjects who had completed the

17

Table 1. Titration Steps Required for Blood Pressure Control.

Patch Strength and No.	No. of Patients
TTS-1	4
TTS-2	2
TTS-3	1
TTS-2 × 2	1
TTS-3 × 2	1

Table 2. Blood Pressure and Pulse in Responders to Transdermal Clonidine.

	Control	Titration (2-6 weeks)	Maintenance (3 + months)
n	9	9	6
Sitting B.P. (mmHg)	$159 \pm 6/98 \pm 1$	$135 \pm 5*/79 \pm 2*$	$129 \pm 8*/73 \pm 3*$
Sitting pulse (beats/minute)	76 ± 3	76 ± 3	75 ± 3
Standing B.P. (mmHg)	$155 \pm 5/93 \pm 2$	$135 \pm 9*/77 \pm 3*$	$123 \pm 10*/67 \pm 3*$
Standing pulse (beats/minute)	74 ± 2	79 ± 2	79 ± 2

* $p < 0.001$ vs control (Student's paired t-test).

maintenance phase of the protocol (Table 2). There were no significant changes in the pulse rates with the transdermal clonidine therapy (Table 2).

Serum electrolytes, complete blood counts, urinalyses, and electrocardiograms did not change significantly at the end of the titration or stable dose phases when compared to the control measurements.

Plasma noradrenaline decreased significantly ($p < 0.05$) from 524 ± 78 at baseline to 334 ± 38 pg/ml in the eight responders in whom it was measured (Fig. 1). The values remained suppressed in three subjects who were studied at the end of three months on a stable dose. No relationship between noradrenaline changes and blood pressure response was found. Plasma adrenaline did not change significantly.

Side-effects: Complaints elicited during the study are listed in Table 3. Mild dry mouth was noted by two subjects and one patient complained of dizziness for one week before evaluation at which time he was found to be mildly hypotensive. One patient had difficulty maintaining the patch in place as he spent a good deal of time in his swimming pool.

The most significant problem was local skin reaction. One subject had very mild itching without inflammation or erythema and this subsided without dosage adjustment. Three other subjects had more significant reactions. One subject had an intense inflammatory response with erythema, oedema and vesiculation at the patch site requiring discontinuation two weeks after the start of active therapy. Two other subjects noted mild irritation in the first few weeks of titration. This became progressively more bothersome with evi-

18

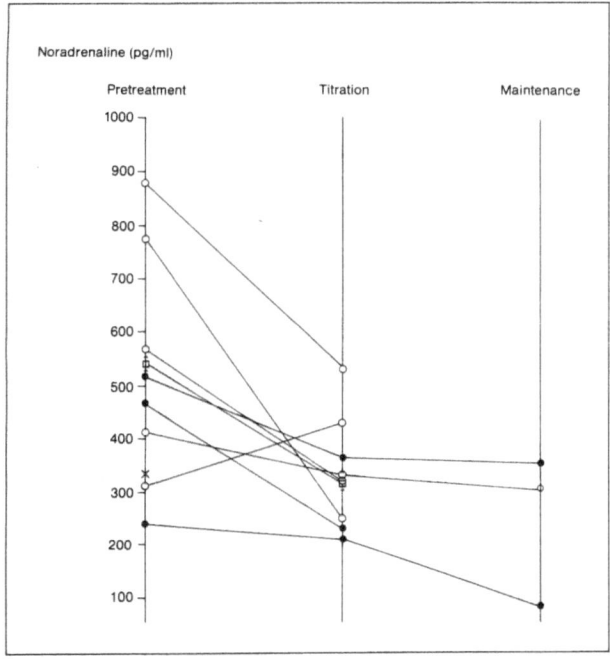

Noradrenaline (pg/ml)

| Pretreatment | Titration | Maintenance |

Fig. 1. Plasma noradrenaline levels at control, end of titration period and at completion of stable dose phase. Closed circles are subjects with skin rash, open circles are patients without rash and x is the single non-responder. ● – skin rash; ○ – no skin rash; x – single non-responder.

Table 3. Side-effects and Complaints During Treatment with Transdermal Clonidine.

Symptom	No. of Patients
Dry mouth-mild	2
Dizziness	1 (Hypotension)
Itching-mild	1
Loss of patch (swimming pool)	1
Skin rash under patch	3

dence of erythema and oedema but without vesiculation. At the end of the stable dose phase neither patient wished to continue using the patches.

Medication Discontinuation: Four subjects were observed after clonidine-TTS discontinuation. Three exhibited a gradual rise to or toward baseline blood pressure levels over a two weeks observation period. One subject who had required the highest dose (two TTS-3) for control during titration phase was found to be hypotensive (B.P. 94/60 mmHg sitting, 75/51 mmHg standing, with a pulse rate of 76 and 78 beats/minute respectively) after three months on this dose. This subject also had skin inflammation and did not wish to continue the protocol. He was told to wear only one patch for four days and then remove it. His next visit was scheduled for three days after removal of the final patch at which time sitting blood pressure was 180/127 mmHg and pulse rate was 83 beats/minute. The patient felt well. The blood pressure remained raised during the following week (187/111 mmHg sitting) despite the addition of nadolol. His blood pressure has subsequently been controlled with a three-drug regimen consisting of nadolol, hydrochlorothiazide and hydralazine.

Discussion

Our experience with clonidine delivered through the skin in elderly subjects with mild hypertension showed both favourable and unfavourable features. Clearly further study with this age group is needed. On one hand 60% of our patients had a good response to the preparation and experienced a very low incidence of side-effects. These subjects were pleased with the convenience of once weekly administration and many are continuing with longer term evaluation. On the other hand one subject did not respond and three experienced significant local skin reactions which would have precluded long-term use. If such a high incidence were to be seen in a larger sample this would present a substantial drawback. One subject had many problems with the use of the system: on the highest dose he eventually became hypotensive; whether this represented a build-up of drug levels is currently being explored. He also experienced a rapid rise in blood pressure after discontinuation although it is now apparent his usual level of blood pressure was more severe than that measured during the placebo period.

Some differences between our experience with oral clonidine therapy and transdermal therapy should be noted. In our previous studies (Thananopavarn et al. 1982) with oral clonidine the suppression of noradrenaline and the slowing of the heart rate both correlated with the effect on blood pressure. In the limited data of the few subjects thus far studied with transdermal clonidine we have confirmed a suppression in plasma noradrenaline levels but did not find a relationship to the blood pressure response. The small number of subjects and the titration regimen which resulted in very uniform blood pressure responses may help to explain this lack of correlation. The failure to demonstrate a slowing of the pulse despite evidence of decreased sympathetic activity in these patients perhaps may be attributed to the decreased responsiveness of chronotropic beta receptors in the elderly. The chronotropic response to clonidine has been attributed to a potentiation of parasympathetic as well as an inhibition of sympathetic mechanisms. The low level of clonidine achieved with the transdermal route could affect these mechanisms differently than the pulsatile blood levels achieved with oral therapy. Finally, the possibility that the route of administration might affect the metabolism of the drug with formation of different active metabolites must be considered.

More experience with the use of transdermal clonidine is needed to clarify its utility and acceptability as monotherapy in mild hypertension and also to understand better its mode of action.

Acknowledgements

The authors thank Dr. N. Vlachakis for performing the catecholamine assay and Ms. P. Walker and Mr. R. Marciano for their clinical assistance.

References

1. Drayer JIM, Weber MA, DeYoung JL, Wyle FA (1982) Circadian blood pressure patterns in ambulatory hypertensive patients. Effects of age. Am J Med 73: 493–499
2. Lakatta EG (1979) Alterations in the cardiovascular system that occur in advanced age. Fed Proc 38: 163–170
3. Sambhi MP (1983) Clonidine monotherapy in mild and moderate hypertension. In Hayduk K and Book KD (eds) Central blood pressure regulation, Steinkopff Verlag, Darmstadt, p 131–142
4. Thananopavarn C, Golub MS, Eggena P, Barrett JD, Sambhi MP (1982) Clonidine, a centrally acting sympathetic inhibitor as monotherapy for mild to moderate hypertension. Am J Card 49: 153–158
5. Thananopavarn C, Golub MS, Sambhi MP (1983) Clonidine in the elderly hypertensive. Monotherapy and therapy with a diuretic. Chest 835: 410S–411S
6. Valchakis ND, Mendlowitz M (1980) Plasma catecholamines in primary hypertension. Biochem Med 23: 35–46
7. Weidmann P, Baretta-Piccoli C, Ziegler WJ et al (1978) Age versus urinary sodium for judging renin, aldosterone and catecholamine levels. Studies in normal subjects and patients with essential hypertension. Kidney Int 14: 619–628

Authors' address:
Mohinder P. Sambhi, M.D.
Division of Hypertension
Sepulveda Veterans Medical Center
16111 Plummer Street
Sepulveda, California 91343
U.S.A.

Effects of Catapres-TTS on Cerebral Blood Flow in Elderly Hypertensive Patients

W. Gary Reed, Michael Devous, Lynne M. Kirk, LaVon Kuhnert,
Carol Matthews, Hazem Chehabi, Ernest Stokeley, Ron J. Anderson, and
Frederick Bonte

Introduction

Hypertension is a major risk factor for certain cardiovascular and cerebrovascular diseases which is present in elderly as well as young patients (Kannel 1974; Shekelle 1974). Treatment of certain hypertensive patients with various hypotensive agents also reduces serious morbidity and mortality (Hypertension Detection and Follow-up Program Cooperative Group 1979). However, antihypertensive therapy may carry a big risk in certain groups of patients, especially the elderly, because the fall in arterial pressure could result in a clinically significant fall in perfusion of certain vital organs such as the brain, kidneys or myocardium (Jackson et al. 1976). Clonidine has been shown to decrease cerebral blood flow when given intravenously to patients with hypertensive emergencies (Bertel et al. 1983), although its effect on regional cerebral blood flow is unknown. Because many elderly hypertensive patients are likely to have subclinical cerebrovascular disease and thus be susceptible to adverse effects of hypotensive therapy, this study was undertaken to examine the effect of clonidine given by a transdermal delivery system on cerebral blood flow in this group. This report summarises the preliminary findings of the effect of Catapres-TTS on cerebral blood flow in elderly patients with mild hypertension.

Methods

Patients at least 60 years old with an untreated diastolic blood pressure of 90–104 mmHg were studied. Patients with significant cardiac, renal, hepatic, metabolic or central nervous system diseases were excluded. Also, patients with a history of depression or alcoholism and those taking barbiturates, tricyclic antidepressants, or phenothiazines were excluded. After a washout placebo phase, diastolic blood pressure was titrated biweekly using Catapres-TTS until the resting diastolic blood pressure was less than 90 mmHg or had fallen by at least 5 mmHg if the baseline diastolic pressure was 90–99 mmHg. If the baseline diastolic pressure was 100–104 mmHg, a 10 mmHg drop in diastolic pressure was required. Cerebral blood flow was measured by a Single Photon Emission Computerised Tomographic (SPECT) method utilising inhaled ^{133}Xe as tracer by the method of

Department of Internal Medicine and Nuclear Medicine Center, University of Texas Health Science Center at Dallas, Southwestern Medical School, Dallas, U.S.A.

Stokeley (1980) at the end of the placebo phase and again one to two weeks after the goal diastolic blood pressure had been reached. Adverse drug effects were determined by patient interviews and physical examinations before and after the titration phase.

Results

Four patients with a mean age of 72 years (66–80 years) and a mean sitting blood pressure of 170/95 mmHg were studied. After titration with Catapres-TTS, mean sitting blood pressure was significantly reduced to 148/87 ($p < 0.05$) utilising Catapres-TTS 3 (7.5 mg clonidine base) in three patients and Catapres-TTS 2 (5 mg clonidine base) in one. No adverse effects were reported or detected in these patients. Changes in mean cerebral blood flow before and after drug therapy are shown in Table 1. In two patients, mean

Table 1. Mean Cerebral Blood Flow in Elderly Patients Treated with Catapres-TTS.

Patient	Cerebral Blood Flow (ml/100 g/min)		
	Placebo		Drug
1	48		39
2	100		78
3	68		71
4	69		68
	71	N.S.	64

N.S. = Not statistically significant ($p = 0.11$)

cerebral blood flow did not change significantly after blood pressure was lowered but in the remaining two it fell. None of the patients experienced symptoms of focal or global cerebral ischaemia. The mean flows of all patients on placebo and Catapres-TTS were 71 ml/100 g/min and 64 ml/100 g/min respectively, but this change was not statistically significant ($p = 0.11$). Mean regional flows also tended to decrease but again, changes were not statistically significant ($p > 0.05$) except in the left parietal region where flow decreased from 84 ml/100 g/min to 73 ml/100 g/min ($p > 0.018$) (Table 2). Changes in systolic, diastolic or mean blood pressure did not correlate with any change in cerebral blood flow. Also, the dose of Catapres-TTS did not correlate with changes in flow.

Discussion

Hypertension is an important factor influencing the incidence of cerebrovascular events regardless of age. The efficacy of antihypertensive therapy in preventing these complications in elderly persons has yet to be conclusively proven. Several studies have suggested that such a benefit may be present and that antihypertensive therapy can be safely undertaken in elderly patients if they are closely monitored (Veterans Administration Cooperative Study 1972).

Table 2. Regional Cerebral Blood Flows in Elderly Patients Treated with Catapres-TTS.

Region	Cerebral Blood Flow (ml/100 g/min)	
	Placebo	Drug
Left Frontal	69	60*
Right Frontal	66	55*
Left Parietal	84	73[+]
Right Parietal	80	74*
Left Temporal	67	62*
Right Temporal	70	59*
Left Inferior Temporal	69	65*
Right Inferior Temporal	73	61*
Left Occipital	75	69*
Right Occipital	78	69*
Cerebellar	72	66*
Left Hemispheric	70	64*
Right Hemispheric	72	65*

* Not statistically significant ($p > 0.05$)
[+] $p = 0.018$

Cerebrovascular disease is very common in elderly persons. Consequently, the effect of antihypertensive drugs on cerebral blood flow is very important in this group. This study was undertaken to examine the effect of clonidine delivered by a transdermal delivery system (Catapres-TTS) on cerebral blood flow in elderly patients without clinically evident neurological impairment.

From these preliminary data, it appears that Catapres-TTS does lower blood pressure in some elderly patients without clinically significant adverse effects. This confirms other studies which have shown the safety of using clonidine in elderly patients with hypertension (Ram et al. 1980).

The effect of clonidine on cerebral blood flow in patients with hypertension has not been extensively studied. Bertel et al. (1983) showed a fall in cerebral blood flow in patients with hypertensive emergencies treated with intravenous clonidine, although the clinical significance of this fall could not be determined. Our data indicate that clonidine delivered by a transdermal delivery system has a variable effect on cerebral blood flow in elderly patients with mild hypertension. Two patients had a significant fall in mean and diastolic blood pressure with no change in cerebral blood flow while two patients with a similar fall in blood pressure experienced a fall in flow, although no clinical effects were demonstrated.

Several reasons exist that could explain the fall in cerebral blood flow seen in some patients treated with clonidine. Clonidine could have a direct effect on cerebral vessels from its α_2-agonistic properties leading to vasoconstriction with a subsequent decrease in flow. Such vasoconstriction, mediated by α_2-adrenoreceptors, has been shown in the forearm of man (Kiowski et al. 1983). Although this mechanism is possible, it seems unlikely because of the two patients who had no change in cerebral blood flow despite a fall in pressure.

Another reason for the fall in cerebral blood flow seen in some patients involves the effect hypertension has on the lower limit of the autoregulation of cerebral blood flow. Several workers (Strandgaard et al. 1973; Barry et al. 1982; Gifford 1983; Fujishima et al. 1984) have convincingly shown that chronic hypertension leads to an upward shift of the auto-regulatory curve for cerebral blood flow. Consequently, patients with chronic hypertension will experience a fall in cerebral blood flow at mean arterial pressure above those tolerated by normotensive persons. However, the pressure at which autoregulation becomes ineffective in hypertensive patients is extremely variable (Strandgaard 1976), as is the position of hypertensive patients on the autoregulatory curve in the untreated state. Consequently, some patients can tolerate a significant reduction in blood pressure without compromising cerebral blood flow, while a similar reduction in blood pressure in other patients will result in a significant fall in cerebral blood flow because the lower limit of autoregulation has been surpassed. A similar effect has been noted with diazoxide, a direct arterial vasodilator, in spontaneously hypertensive rats (Barry et al. 1983), where a significant fall in cerebral blood flow was observed if mean arterial blood pressure was lowered to a level below the lower limit of autoregulation. This was felt to be a consequence of the fall in blood pressure to a level below the lower limit of autoregulation and not due to a direct effect of the drug or a loss of autoregulatory function. A similar explanation may account for the observed fall in cerebral blood flow in some of our patients, i.e., the blood pressure was lowered beyond the lower limit of effective autoregulation. The exact mechanism responsible for the fall in cerebral blood flow seen in some patients treated with clonidine, however, remains unknown and further studies are needed to clarify this observation.

In summary, clonidine delivered by a transdermal delivery system (Catapres-TTS) appears to be an effective means to lower blood pressure without serious side effects in elderly patients with mild hypertension. Hypotensive therapy with this agent in elderly hypertensive patients has a variable effect on cerebral blood flow. Further studies should determine whether the changes observed are clinically significant.

Acknowledgement

This study was supported by a grant from Boehringer Ingelheim Ltd.

References

1. Barry DI, Strandgaard S, Graham DI, Braendstrup O, Svendsen UG, Vorstrup S, Hemmingsen R, Bolwig TG (1982) Cerebral blood flow in rats with renal and spontaneous hypertension: resetting of the lower limit of autoregulation. Journal of Cerebral Blood Flow and Metabolism 2: 347–353
2. Barry DI, Strandgaard S, Graham DI, Braendstrup O, Svendsen UG, Bolwig TG (1983) Effect of diazoxide-induced hypotension on cerebral blood flow in hypertensive rats. Eur J Clin Invest 13: 201–207
3. Bertel O, Conen D, Radü EW, Müller J, Lang C, Duback UC (1983) Nifedipine in hypertensive emergencies. Br Med J 286: 19–21
4. Fujishima M, Sadoshima S, Ogata J, Yoshida F, Shiokawa O, Ibayashi S, Omae T (1984) Autoregulation of cerebral blood flow in young and aged spontaneously hypertensive rats. Gerontology 30: 30–36
5. Gifford RW, Jr (1983) Effect of reducing elevated blood pressure on cerebral circulation. Hypertension 5 (Suppl III) III-17–III-20

6. Hypertension Detection and Follow-up Program Cooperative Group (1979) Five-year Findings of the Hypertension Detection and Follow-up Program. II. Mortality by race, sex, and age. JAMA 242: 2572–2577
7. Jackson G, Pierscianowski TA, Mahon W, Condon J (1976) Inappropriate antihypertensive therapy in the elderly. Lancet 2; 1317–1318
8. Kannel WB (1974) Role of blood pressure in cardiovascular morbidity and mortality. Prog Cardiovasc Dis 17: 5–24
9. Kiowski W, Hulthen UL, Ritz R, Bühler FR (1983) α_2 Adrenoceptor-mediated vasoconstriction of arteries. Clin Pharmacol Ther 34: 565–569
10. Mackenzie ET, Strandgaard S, Graham DI, Jones JV, Harper AM, Farrar K (1976) Effects of acutely induced hypertension in cats on pial arteriolar caliber, local cerebral blood flow and the blood brain barrier. Circ Res 39: 33–39
11. Ram CVS, Anderson RJ, Hart GR, Kaplan NM (1980) Assessment of blood pressure control during once-a-day administration of antihypertensive drugs. Curr Ther Res 28: 88–95
12. Shekelle RB, Ostfeld AM, Klawans HL (1974) Hypertension and risk of stroke in an elderly population. Stroke 5: 71–75
13. Stokeley EM, Sveinsdottir E, Lassen NA, Rommer P (1980) A single photon dynamic computer assisted tomograph (DCAT) for imaging brain function in multiple cross sections. A Comput Assist Tomogr 4: 230–240
14. Strandgaard S, Olesen, J, Skinhoj E, Lassen NA (1973) Autoregulation of brain circulation in severe arterial hypertension. Br Med J I: 507–509
13. Strandgaard S (1976) Autoregulation of cerebral blood flow in hypertensive patients. The modifying influence of prolonged antihypertensive treatment on the tolerance to acute, drug-induced hypotension. Circulation 53: 720–727
16. Veterans Administration Cooperative Study Group on Antihypertensive Agents (1972) Effects of treatment on morbidity in hypertension. III. Influence of age, diastolic pressure and prior cardiovascular disease: further analysis of side effects. Circulation 45: 991–1004

Authors' address:
W. Gary Reed, M.D.
Department of Internal Medicine
and Nuclear Medicine Center
University of Texas Health Science
5323 Harry Hines Boulevard
Dallas, Texas 75235
U.S.A.

Discussion

MATHIAS:

I should like to ask Dr. Bravo a question. During your talk, I had the impression that the plasma nor-adrenaline levels in most of your patients were not grossly elevated. If you use this measurement as an index of peripheral sympathetic nervous activity, can you really conclude that there is evidence of increased sympathetic nervous activity in hypertension? Would it not be more accurate to say that there is an inappropriately sustained elevation of sympathetic nervous activity? This broader concept allows the possibility that mechanisms distal to the sympathetic nerve endings, such as receptors, might play a major role?

BRAVO:

We found that patients whose plasma concentrations of noradrenaline were 250 pg/ml or higher had clearly greater antihypertensive responses to treatment with clonidine than patients whose values were 250 pg/ml or lower. Thus, there did appear to be some evidence for an enhanced level of sympathetic nervous system activity in those patients who had the greatest response to clonidine.

MATHIAS:

Does this mean that you believe that there are subgroups within the hypertensive population?

BRAVO:

I think that is a reasonable assumption. Several investigators have shown that about 30% of hypertensive patients may be hyperadrenergic.

SOWERS:

I should like to ask Dr. Anlauf whether there is a relationship between α_2-receptors and plasma nor-adrenaline levels?

ANLAUF:

We have not as yet directly measured the relationship in hypertensive patients between plasma nor-adrenaline and the number of α_2-receptors, but we believe that there is an increase in both. This suggests that perhaps in hypertension we have a defect in the regulation of these receptors.

CALNAN:

I am interested in the description of the skin rashes reported by Dr. Sambhi in his study. Does your diagnosis of rash mean a reaction at the patch site only, or does it also mean skin lesions at any other site?

27

SAMBHI:

We did not see any generalized skin rashes in any of our patients. The skin reactions that we saw were strictly limited to the area under the patch. From a clinical point of view, we tended to classify the rash into two categories. In two of our patients, it was a simple erythaematous reaction associated with mild pruritis and was reported to be reasonably tolerable. In another patient, the rash was categorized by vesiculations and we had to discontinue the treatment. However, even in this more severe case, the skin reaction occurred only under the area of the patch and was not generalized.

SOWERS:

Dr. Reed, from your studies, do you think that α_2-stimulation by clonidine could actually increase cerebral blood flow rather than decrease it?

REED:

The role of the α_2-receptors in the vessels of the cerebral circulation has not yet been fully defined. However, in studies of forearm peripheral blood flow, it has been shown that stimulation of the α_2-receptor has produced a decrease in blood flow, but it is possible that these receptors may mediate differing physiological functions in the central and peripheral arterial circulations.

MANCIA:

In his presentation, Dr. Bravo has dealt with an old but important controversy. How reliable is the measurement of plasma noradrenaline concentration as an index of sympathetic tone, and can we use the presence of increased plasma concentrations of noradrenaline as evidence for heightened sympathetic activity? I believe it is important to be very cautious in making such interpretations; firstly, less than 1% of noradrenaline secreted from the sympathetic neurons actually spills over into the plasma. Secondly, it is likely that there are differences between the various vascular beds and that the overall plasma noradrenaline concentration therefore does not give us a balanced view of the various interactions between the sympathetic nervous system and the cardiovascular system. There are other factors which also determine the levels of plasma noradrenaline. For example, it has been shown that the clearance of noradrenaline is reduced in elderly subjects and this may account for the raised plasma noradrenaline concentrations that are found in these individuals. Thus, the claims that have been made that there is sympathetic overactivity in elderly patients may be based on a questionable assumption. Another method which has been used to assess sympathetic function in hypertensive patients is by measuring the responsiveness to sympatholytic drugs. However, these kind of data are also difficult to interpret because these agents have several mechanisms of action and we cannot be certain that their effectiveness in lowering blood pressure reflects their ability to block sympathetic mechanisms. The matter is made even more confusing by the likelihood that hypertensive patients have highly variable responses to sympathetic stimuli. Responses to sympathetic stimuli such as handgrip tests or the cold pressor test are not always reproducible, and the relationships between such tests is not always predictable. Thus, again, it is difficult to be certain just how important measurements of the sympathetic nervous system at rest, or even during stimulated conditions, can be in estimating the actual contribution of sympathetic factors to the hypertension.

BRAVO:

I agree with Dr. Mancia that great care is required in using measurements of circulating catecholamines as an index of sympathetic tone. I also agree that it may be difficult to accurately interpret the significance of the blood pressure-lowering actions of the various sympatholytic drugs. Nevertheless, I believe that there is a reasonable degree of specificity in the effects of centrally-acting agents such as clonidine. Moreover, we have had now a long experience with these types of agents in the treatment of patients with hypertension, and there is quite strong evidence indicating that they tend to be most effective in those patients in whom there is evidence for increased sympathetic activity, usually increased plasma noradrenaline; thus, while I agree with the important comments that Dr. Mancia has put forward, I still believe that the assumptions we have made concerning the sympathetic nervous system and its role in hypertension are valid.

KRAFT:

I should like to ask Professor Anlauf whether he has performed animal or in vitro studies to determine the number and sensitivity of α_2-receptors simultaneously in tissues and in platelets. Is there a positive correlation between these measurements in platelets and in other tissues?

ANLAUF:

The studies we have reported here were based on human investigation, and I cannot answer your question directly. Studies performed by other investigators to look at this issue have provided inconsistent results, perhaps reflecting differences between species. I agree with Dr. Kraft, however, that it would be important to do further comparisons of α_2-receptor density in thrombocytes and other tissues.

FERDER:

The skin findings reported by Dr. Sambhi were very interesting. Is there any way of predicting which patients might have skin reactions to the transdermal medication? For example, does the colour of the skin, or perhaps the degree of hair growth, indicate the likelihood of such a reaction?

SAMBHI:

In our relatively limited experience we have not seen any predictable indicators of likely skin reactions. The three patients who developed reactions during our study did experience some irritation during the first week of treatment. However, as I remarked earlier, two of these three patients continued to the end of the study without being especially inconvenienced by the skin effects.

WEBER:

Antihypertensive drugs that work primarily in the central nervous system can produce side-effects such as drowsiness or depression. Dr. Reed, did you find any relationship between changes in cerebral blood flow and the presence of these types of symptoms?

REED:

I think that there is a relationship between decreases in cerebral blood flow and the onset of drowsiness. However, this is probably not a major factor in the clinical symptoms which we usually find during antihypertensive treatment. In the studies that I presented here we did not find any correlation between the appearance of drowsiness and changes in cerebral blood flow.

GUTHRIE:

Did any of the patients reported by Dr. Bravo have clinically overt signs or symptoms of excessive sympathetic tone? As you know, there have been reports of patients with so-called hyperkinetic hearts of pseudo-phaeochromocytoma in which there are findings such as sweatiness and tachycardia. In your experience, do such patients show a particularly good response to treatment with agents such as clonidine?

BRAVO:

Only one of our patients in the present study appeared to have a hyperkinetic syndrome. However, we have treated several patients with hyperkinetic findings and pseudo-phaeochromocytoma symptoms, and in our experience, these patients respond well to clonidine. It is interesting, however, that the plasma catecholamine concentrations in these patients are not always very high. It is possible that these individuals have heightened vascular sensitivity to sympathetic effects or that the increases in sympathetic activity occur only during the clinical symptoms and are not found at other times. This apparent lack of association between plasma catecholamine measurements and clinical findings is in agreement with the comments made earlier by Dr. Mancia.

SAMBHI:

Professor Anlauf has reported that the density of α_2-receptors is increased in hypertensive individuals. I should like to ask him two brief questions. First, is it possible that this increase in receptor density could be due directly to the rise in blood pressure itself? And secondly, have you studied α_2-receptor density in normotensive relatives of hypertensive patients?

ANLAUF:

We have investigated patients with phaeochromocytoma who have had high plasma concentrations of catecholamines, and have found that they actually had a down regulation of their α_2-receptors. It is not possible to be certain whether this finding reflects changes in blood pressure or whether it simply reflects a reaction to the hormone itself. Your question about receptor density in the normotensive relatives of hypertensive patients is an important one, and it is presently being studied.

Lipid Metabolism and Antihypertensive Treatment

C. Diehm and H. Mörl

Introduction

There have recently been more references in the literature to plasma lipid changes during antihypertensive treatment. Interest in these drug-induced changes in lipid metabolism is increasing, together with the question of whether they predispose to atherosclerosis. The changes in lipoproteins induced by antihypertensive drugs are of clinical interest, as epidemiological data indicate that a decrease in high-density lipoprotein cholesterol fractions (HDL cholesterol), which are protective, and increases in low-density lipoprotein cholesterol fractions (LDL cholesterol) are associated with an increased risk of coronary heart disease (Miller and Miller 1975; Castelli 1977; Taggart and Stout 1979; Glynn et al. 1982; Rössner 1982) (Tables 1–4).

Table 1. Importance of High-Density Lipoprotein (HDL) cholesterol.

	HDL Cholesterol (mg/dl)
Risk indicator	< 35
Grey zone	35–55
Prognostically favourable	> 55

Table 2. Rating of Low-density Lipoprotein (LDL) Cholesterol.

	LDL Cholesterol (mg/dl)
Ideal	< 150
Transitional range	150–190
Intervention level	> 190

Table 3. Factors Leading to a Reduction in High-density Lipoprotein Cholesterol.

- Obesity (at the present time still controversial)
- Cigarette smoking
- Oral contraceptives
- Male as compared to female
- Diabetes mellitus
- Coronary heart disease
- Cerebrovascular disease
- Peripheral vascular disease
- Hyperlipoproteinaemia Types II, IV and V

Medizinische Universitätsklinik Heidelberg, F.R.G.

Table 4. Factors that Raise the Plasma HDL-Cholesterol Concentration.

Oestrogens	Gustafson and Svanburg 1972
	Bradley et al. 1978
Alcohol	Johansson and Laurell 1966
	Hulley et al. 1977
	Castelli et al. 1977
Physical endurance training	Wood et al. 1976
	Lehtonen and Viikari 1978
Heparin infusions	Nikkilä 1978
Bezafibrate	Olson and Lang 1978
Nicotinic acid derivates	Blum et al. 1977
Phenytoin and phenobarbitone	Nikkilä et al. 1978
Chlorinated hydrocarbon	Carlson and Kolomodin-Hedman
Compounds (insecticides)	Compounds
Familial high-density Lipoproteinaemia	Glück et al. 1975

Diuretics and impaired fat metabolism

Most of the studies were carried out with medium to high doses of thiazide diuretics; they show that in young and elderly men with hypertension and in women in the post-menopause, diuretics do not increase total cholesterol and low-density lipoproteins (LDL) are only increased slightly, by 8–10%, while the triglyceride and very low density lipoprotein levels (VLDL) can increase much more i.e. 10–28%. The high density lipoproteins (HDL) usually remain unaffected (Ames and Hill 1976; Glück et al. 1980; Johnson 1982; Weidmann et al. 1983; Krone et al. 1984; Zumkley et al. 1984).
These effects have been found with all diuretics so far investigated, including those acting on Henle's loop. These changes are also attributed to the newer loop-active diuretics of the muzolimine type (Schiffl et al. 1984). The only exception is one of the newer diuretic-antihypertensive agents, indapamide, which does not cause any significant rise in the plasma LDL cholesterol (Weidmann et al. 1981), chlorthalidone is another diuretic likely to produce adverse changes in lipoproteins. The failure to make simultaneous analyses of the different lipoprotein fractions made it difficult to interpret the first reports of increases in triglycerides and total cholesterol in the course of diuretic treatment (Ames and Hill 1976; Schnaper et al. 1977). Changes in plasma LDL levels which occurred in the course of diuretic treatment did not correlate with changes in blood pressure, body weight, or plasma potassium level, nor were they associated with changes in the plasma glucose and insulin levels (Weidmann et al. 1981). Altogether there are no indications of the basic mechanisms responsible for the changes in lipoproteins during treatment with diuretics. It is important, however, that in many of the studies the investigators failed to take account of changes in diet or body weight during the investigation. Most failed to correlate the lipoprotein fractions with the relevant haematocrit and blood protein levels. Furthermore, no attention was paid to the changes in haemoconcentration associated

with diuretic treatment, especially in the initial stages. The period of the study was often too short.

According to recent studies low but effective doses of hydrochlorothiazide or chlorthalidone (15–25 mg/day) do not affect the lipids even over a lengthy period of time (Zumkley et al. 1984). Since diuretics are used as step-one products for the treatment of high blood pressure low doses should be given, with another drug if greater effect is required.

β-Blockers and lipoprotein changes

Lipoprotein concentrations have been shown to be adversely affected by monotherapy with β-adrenergic blocking agents (Waal-Manning 1976; Bielmann and Leduc 1979; Leren et al. 1982; Lohmann 1983) such as propranalol and the cardioselective metoprolol. β-receptor blockers without cardioselectivity and without intrinsic sympathomimetic action (ISA) have shown the poorest results. After propranolol total triglycerides rose by 20–60% with a corresponding rise in VLDL. The total cholesterol and LDL were only slightly affected, while HDL were occasionally slightly reduced. Cardioselective β-blockers and β-blockers with ISA show the same effect on fat metabolism, but to a lesser degree (Eliason et al. 1981; Franz et al. 1984; Krone et al. 1984) (Fig. 1).

It is not clear how the β-blockers cause changes in lipid metabolism, the effects of β-blockers on lipolysis may play a major part. When β-blockers are given alone, increased α-activity may raise the triglyceride levels by inhibition or the lipoprotein lipase (Fig. 1). Thus it is important that nonselective β-blockers are more potent than cardioselective agents in inhibiting lipolysis (Sitori et al. 1982). At present we cannot assess the clinical importance of biochemical findings associated with β-receptor blockade. Clinical experience, however, shows that the therapeutic value of the β-blockers, used in response to the appropriate indications, outweighs any atherogenic effects. β_1-selective adrenergic blocking agents have fewer adverse effects on the lipoproteins and should therefore be preferred, even in patients with primary hyperlipoproteinaemia. By contrast, some long-

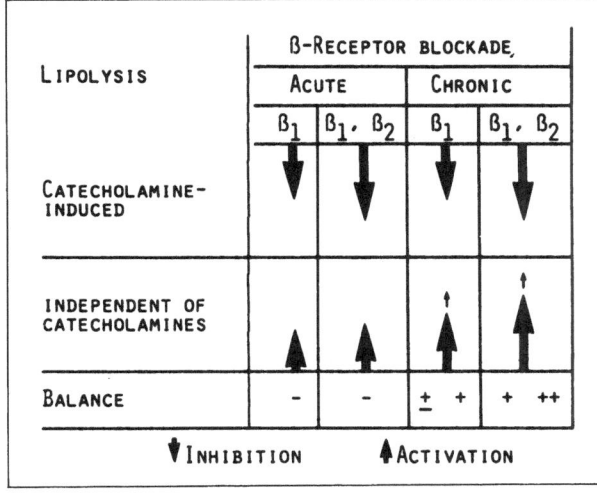

Fig. 1. Effects of β-blockade on lipolysis.

term studies, in which the behaviour of the plasma lipids in response to β-receptor blockade was followed for up to six years, showed that there may not be any relevant changes in the lipoproteins (Schnaper et al. 1977; Kristensen 1981). These studies included reductions in body weight in association with a patient care system, and the patients also achieved improved glucose tolerance. Long-term studies are required to permit a final evaluation of the clinical validity of these responses to β-receptor blockade.

Prazosin and lipoprotein mechanism

In several studies the total cholesterol, triglyceride and thus the LDL and VLDL levels were reduced with prazosin treatment, but the HDL level increased (Kirkendall 1978; Leren et al. 1982). The "Oslo study" showed treatment with prazosin for eight weeks reduced the LDL and the VLDL cholesterol levels, as well as the total triglycerides; however, treatment with propranolol over the same period resulted in a marked decrease in HDL cholesterol (Leren et al. 1982). Pindolol and hydrochlorothiazide had no effect; atenolol administered for five weeks slightly reduced the LDL and the VLDL cholesterol levels, and oxprenolol raised the triglyceride levels. Prazosin plus pindolol was the most advantageous combination of antihypertensive agents. However, the study period was short and each group consisted of only 10–33 subjects, which detracts from the validity of this study. Furthermore, patients with marked hyper-β-lipoproteinaemia were over represented in the sample.

Vasodilator antihypertensives and lipoprotein metabolism

High doses of hydralazine lower the total cholesterol according to an older study. The effect on the various lipid fractions has not been investigated to date.
No controlled studies have been carried out on the effects of calcium antagonists on these serum lipid levels.

Clonidine and lipoprotein metabolism

In a comparative study clonidine lowered the overall cholesterol level to the same extent as prazosin (Kirkendall et al. 1978). We examined the effect of clonidine ("Catapres") on the lipoprotein fractions in the serum in a pilot study.

Patients and Methods

Twelve male outpatients aged between 48 and 72 years (average age 57.0 ± 7.3 years) participated in the study. All the patients had essential hypertension of which they had been aware for one to 10 years and which had previously been treated with other antihypertensives. Five patients also had coronary heart disease, four patients arterial occlusion, one patient primary chronic polyarthritis and one patient hypertrophy of the prostate and a duodenal ulcer. Antihypertensive therapy was discontinued 14 days before the start of the Catapres study, and the necessary concomitant therapy maintained at a constant dosage during the washout phase and treatment with clonidine. Catapres was given for 12 weeks in doses of 2×0.075 mg to 3×0.150 mg (mean: 0.244 mg) per day.

The blood pressure and pulse rate were measured in the washout phase at seven-day intervals, and at four-week intervals during therapy with Catapres, in a supine and standing position. The serum lipoproteins examined from various angles by means of ultracentrifugation were monitored every four weeks as were other blood-chemical values such as fasting blood sugar, sodium potassium and uric acid in the serum, and liver enzymes.

The changes in blood pressure and pulse rate were evaluated by means of variance analysis. A Wilcoxon pair difference test was carried out for the lipoproteins (before clonidine compared with after 12 weeks' clonidine treatment) with stratification. The other laboratory parameters were examined by the Friedman test.

Results

As of the end of the preliminary period the blood pressure fell significantly, in a supine position, from $186.7 \pm 8.6/102.9 \pm 7.2$ mmHg to $151.3 \pm 5.3/91.7 \pm 7.2$ mmHg after 12 weeks' clonidine therapy. Values measured in a standing position showed barely any differences compared with those in a supine position (Fig. 2).

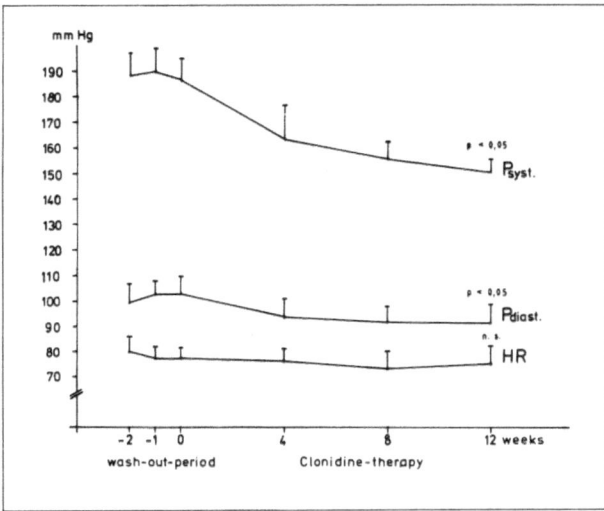

Fig. 2. Blood pressure and heart rate before and after four, eight and twelve weeks on clonidine therapy. (Mean values $\pm$ SD, $n = 12$.)

At the end of the preliminary period the pulse rate was 76.7 ± 4.7 beats per minute, after 12 weeks' clonidine therapy 75.3 ± 7.3 beats per minute in a supine position. There was no statistically significant change in pulse rate after clonidine either in a supine position or standing (Fig. 3).

With clonidine therapy the total cholesterol fell from 240.53 ± 17.4 to 233.95 ± 11.99 mg%, but this change is not significant. In the same 12 week period the triglyceride level dropped from 148.75 ± 48.13 to 140.88 ± 35.0 mg% (not significant). The HDL-

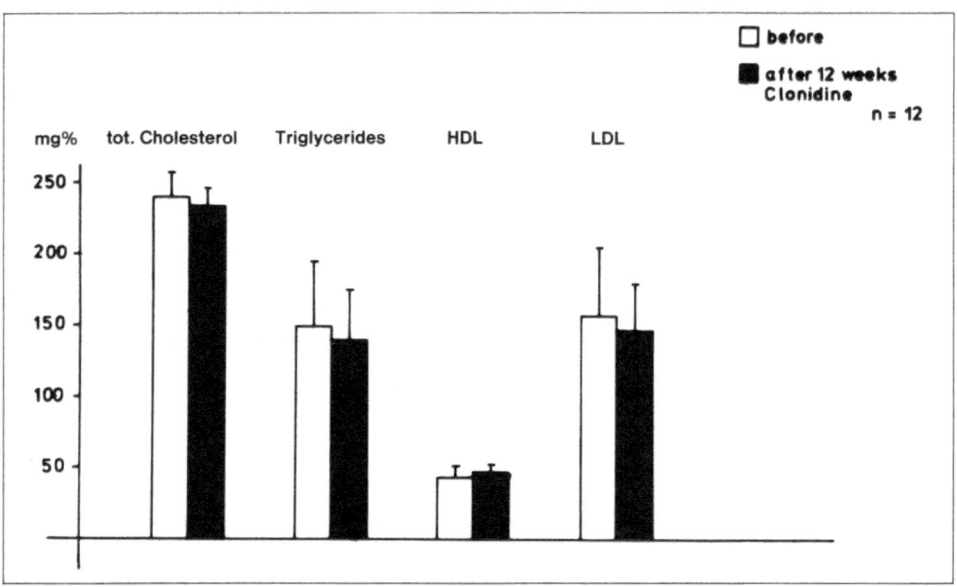

Fig. 3. Total cholesterol, triglycerides, high-density lipoproteins (HDL) and low-density lipoproteins (LDL) before and after twelve weeks' clonidine. (Mean values ± SD, n = 12.)

cholesterol level tended to rise from 44.08 ± 7.30 to 46.92 ± 5.48 mg% after 12 week's treatment with clonidine, while the LDL-cholesterol level tended to drop from 158.17 ± 48.37 to 147.08 ± 32.47 mg%.

Body weight fell during the 12 week clonidine treatment period, without any dietetic measures, from 82.50 ± 9.38 kg to 78.92 ± 8.85 kg (p < 0.001).

In patients with high initial HDL-cholesterol values (> 48 mg%) clonidine had no effect, while in patients with low initial HDL-cholesterol values (> 42 mg%, n = 6) there was on average an increase from 37.6 mg% to 43.7 mg% (p > 0.05). On the other hand, patients with high initial LDL-cholesterol values (> 160 mg%, n = 5) reacted with an average drop from 195 mg% to 165 mg% after clonidine (p < 0.05).

In the other laboratory tests there were no changes after clonidine therapy except for the sodium level in the serum which was found to have fallen after four and eight weeks therapy (p > 0.05) but had risen again on the next check at the end of the 12th week of therapy to the original value (Tables 5 and 6).

Conclusions

The changes in lipoprotein metabolism described with diuretics and β-receptor blockers are usually not so serious that they must be used with great caution. With the β-receptor blockers the benefit outweighs the minimal risk because of the changes in fat metabolism, which is why the dose should not be increased (Zumkley et al. 1984). The problem of changes in fat metabolism, however, in long-term treatment of mild hypertension in young patients should be noted. It is still unclear whether lipid-neutral antihypertensive would be beneficial in this situation.

Table 5. Laboratory tests before and after clonidine treatment. (Mean values $\pm$ SD, n = 12.)

	Before	Treatment with Clonidine		
		After 4 weeks	8 weeks	12 weeks
Haemoglobin (mmol/l)	9.3 ± 0.40	9.26 ± 0.76	9.32 ± 0.53	9.42 ± 0.38
Haematocrit (1)	0.44 ± 0.03	0.46 ± 0.06	0.45 ± 0.05	0.44 ± 0.03
Serum-Na$^+$ (mmol/l)	142.00 ± 2.73	$140.25 \pm 3.19*$	$139.25 \pm 3.55*$	142.33 ± 2.10
Serum-potassium (mmol/l)	3.94 ± 0.25	4.02 ± 0.34	4.10 ± 0.31	4.02 ± 0.20
SGOT (U/l)	17.17 ± 5.08	18.17 ± 4.30	17.83 ± 3.24	16.25 ± 2.83
SGPT (U/l)	17.33 ± 5.90	17.67 ± 4.58	17.17 ± 4.47	17.50 ± 4.01
Gamma-GT (U/l)	28.83 ± 11.82	24.00 ± 6.38	25.00 ± 9.78	22.33 ± 6.02
Alkaline phosphatase (U/l)	133.92 ± 24.79	127.42 ± 27.28	126.92 ± 22.90	130.08 ± 15.82
Uric acid (μmol/l)	397.52 ± 53.13	401.99 ± 46.17	386.62 ± 50.34	381.17 ± 49.92
Urea-N (mmol/l)	6.24 ± 1.97	6.99 ± 2.29	6.34 ± 1.87	6.78 ± 1.71
Fasting serum-glucose (mmol/l)	5.06 ± 0.78	5.17 ± 0.87	5.06 ± 0.67	5.18 ± 0.58
Serum-creatinine (μmol/l)	98.71 ± 10.55	90.61 ± 15.60	96.50 ± 14.82	102.40 ± 10.96

$*$ $p < 0.05$.

Table 6. Changes of the Lipoprotein-concentrations After Treatment with Antihypertensives.

Drug Groups	Effect on				
	TG	CHOL	VLDL	LDL	HDL
Thiazide-diuretics				=	
Frusemide		=		=	=
Spironolactone	=	=	?	=	
β-Blockers		=		=	
Prazosin					
Clonidine			?		

References

1. Ames RP, Hill P (1976) Elevation of serum lipid levels during diuretic therapy of hypertension. Am J Med 61: 748–757
2. Bielmann P, Leduc G (1979) Effects of metoprolol and propranolol on lipid metabolism. Int J Clin Pharmac Biopharm 17: 378–382
3. Castelli WP (1977) High density lipoproteins: a new understanding of cholesterol and risk. Am Heart Associations Fourth Science Writers Forum San Antonio Texas
4. Day JL, Metcalfe J, Simpson CN (1982) Adrenergic mechanisms in control of plasma lipid concentrations. Br Med J 284: 1145–1148
5. Eliason K. Lins LE, Rössner S (1981) Serum lipoprotein changes during atenolol treatment of essential hypertension. Eur J Clin Pharmacol 20: 335–338

6. England JDF, Simons LA, Gibson JC, Carlton M (1980) The effect of metoprolol and atenolol on plasma high density lipoprotein levels in man. Clin Exp Pharmacol Physiol 7: 329

7. Franz JW, Lohmann FW, Röcker L (1984) Unterschiedlicher Einfluß einer Langzeittherapie mit β_1-selektiven und β_1-β_2-Rezeptorenblockern auf den Lipidstoffwechsel bei Hochdruckkranken. Herz/Kreislauf 3: 115–122

8. Glück Z, Weidmann P, Mordasini R et al (1980) Increased serum low density lipoprotein cholesterol in men treated short-term with the diuretic chlorthalidone. Metabolism 29: 240–245

9. Glynn RJ, Rosner B, Silbert JE (1982) Changes in cholesterol and triglyceride as predictors of ischemic heart disease in men. Circulation 66: 724–731

10. Johnson BF (1982) The emerging problem of plasma lipid changes during antihypertensive therapy. J of Cardiovasc Pharmacol 4: 213–221

11. Kirkendall WM, Hammond JJ, Thomas JC, Overturf ML, Zama A (1978) Prazosin and clonidine for moderately severe hypertension. JAMA 23: 2553–2556

12. Kristensen BO (1981) Effect of long-term treatment with beta-blocking drugs on plasma lipids and lipoproteins. Br Med J 283: 191

13. Krone W, Müller-Wieland D, Greten H (1984) Antihypertensive Therapie und Fettstoffwechsel. Klin Wochenschr 62: 193–202

14. Leren P, Eide OP, Foss A, Helgeland I, Jermann IH, Holme I, Kjeldsen SE, Lund-Larsen PG (1982) Antihypertensive drugs and blood lipids: The Oslo Study. J of Cardiovasc Pharmacol Vol. 4 Raven Press New York

15. Lohmann FW, Schettler G, Mörl H, Lohmann FW, Wirth A (1983) Serum-Lipidveränderungen durch Beta-Blocker: Metabolische und kardioprotektive Effekte durch Beta-Rezeptoren-Blockade. Springer-Verlag Berlin–Heidelberg–New York–Tokyo

16. Meiser AP, Weidman R, Mordasini R et al (in press) Reversal or prevention of diuretic-induced alterations in serum lipoproteins with betablockers. Atherosclerosis

17. Miettinen TA, Huttunen JK, Ehnholm Chr, Kumlin T, Mattila S, Naukkarinen V (1980) Effect of long-term antihypertensive and hypolipidemic treatment on high density lipoprotein cholesterol and apolipoproteins A-I and A-II. Atherosclerosis 36: 249

18. Miller EJ, Miller NE (1975) Plasma high density lipoprotein concentration and development of ischemic heart disease. Lancet 1: 16

19. Rössner S (1982) Serum lipoproteins and ischemic vascular disease: on the interpretation of serum lipid versus serum lipoprotein concentrations. J of Cardiovasc Pharmacol 4: 201–205

20. Schiffl H, Boehringer K, Weidmann P et al (in press) Effects of diuretic muzolimine on serum lipoproteins

21. Schnaper H, Fitz A, Fröchl E et al. (1977) Chlorthalidone and serum cholesterol. Lancet 2: 295

22. Sitori CR, Shoeman DW, Azarnoff DL (1972) Dissociation of the metabolic and cardiovascular effects of the β-adrenergic blocker practolol. Pharmacol Res Commun 4: 123–133

23. Taggart H, Stout RW (1979) Reduced high density lipoprotein in stroke: relationship with elevated triglyceride and hypertension. Eur J of Clin Invest 9: 219–221

24. Waal-Manning HJ (1976) Metabolic effects of β-adrenoceptor blockers. Drugs 11: (Suppl 1) 121

25. Weidmann P, Meier A, Mordasini R et al (1981) Diuretic treatment and serum lipoproteins: effect of tienilic acid and indapamide. Klin Wochenschr 59: 343–346

26. Weidmann P, Schiffl H, Boehringer K, Meier A, Mordasini R, Riesen W, Glück Z, Beretta-Piccoli C (1981) Einfluß von Diuretika allein oder in Kombination mit Beta-Blockern auf die Serum-Lipoproteine. In: Krück F, Schrey A (Eds) Diuretika II Wolf & Sohn Verlag Munich: 254–273

27. Weidmann P, Gerber A, Mordasini R (1983) Effects of antihypertensive therapy on serum lipoproteins. Hypertension 5/5 Supp III: 120–131

28. Zumkley H, Losse H, Vetter H, Assmann G, Raidt H, Böhmann C, Karoff CH, Baumgart P (in press) Lipidstoffwechsel unter Saluretika-Therapie. Münch Med Wochenschr.

Authors' address:
PD Dr. C. Diehm
Medizinische Universitätsklinik
Bergheimer Straße 58
6900 Heidelberg
F.R.G.

Diabetes and Hypertension: Clonidine Monotherapy

Gordon P. Guthrie, Jr.

Introduction

Hypertension and diabetes mellitus frequently occur together. Half of all diabetics may eventually become hypertensive (Christlieb 1973), most developing so-called essential hypertension partly related to the frequent occurrence of obesity in the diabetic population, and also perhaps reflecting relative expansion of the extracellular fluid space (de Chatel et al. 1977) or poor compliance of large vessels in turn producing high systolic blood pressures. Usually, however, hypertension in diabetics is related to the development of diabetic nephropathy and the characteristic glomerular lesion. Other possible mechanisms are large vessel atherosclerosis leading to renovascular hypertension (Muichoodappa et al. 1979) and abnormalities in diabetic neural function (and perhaps the baroreflex) leading to a rise in supine blood pressure.

Hypertension in the diabetic patient has several important implications. Both hypertension and diabetes produce microvascular and macrovascular damage, seen as damage to the microcirculation of the eye, brain, kidney and other organs, and as atherosclerosis, with consequent risk for stroke and myocardial infarction. Current evidence suggests that these independent effects are augmented when they occur in the same patient. Also, several studies have revealed that when a hypertensive diabetic has his blood pressure effectively controlled, the progression of diabetic retinopathy (Knowler et al. 1980) and nephropathy (Mogenson 1982) is slowed. Therefore, effective control of raised blood pressure in the diabetic patient has special importance.

Recent controlled clinical trials have shown a small, but significant, reduction in cardiovasar morbidity and mortality produced by treating uncomplicated mild hypertension in non-diabetic patients (HDFP 1979). However, whether these results can be universally applied to the treatment of the many patients with asymptomatic, uncomplicated mild hypertension remains undecided (Toth and Horwitz 1983). However, given the increased risk of mild hypertension with diabetics, hypertension of any degree of severity is probably best treated in diabetic patients.

Before drug treatment, other approaches to the treatment of both hypertension and diabetes might be attempted in certain patients. Several studies, some well controlled, have shown that reduction of dietary salt intake to less than 100 mEq/day can reduce blood pressure in some hypertensive patients (MacGregor et al. 1982). Although such favourable blood pressure responses can be idiosyncratic and limited to so-called salt-sensitive individuals, such attempts to limit dietary salt intake to moderate amounts might be attempted in patients receptive to such intervention. Efforts to reduce the weight of the

Department of Medicine, University of Kentucky College of Medicine, Lexington, Kentucky, U.S.A.

obese hypertensive diabetic patient should clearly be initiated for several reasons. Obesity induces both glucose intolerance and hypertension specific for the obese state (Messerli 1982), and both diseases may respond to effective weight loss. In addition, the cardiovascular demands produced by obesity can be serious in such patients. Conditioning isotonic exercise has been reported both to increase insulin sensitivity and glucose tolerance in Type II diabetics, and to produce favourable effects on blood pressure in less well controlled trials (Krotkiewski et al. 1979). Finally, modifications of other nutrients than salt including potassium, fibre content of the diet, and calcium supplementation have been shown in preliminary studies to favourably effect blood pressure. Such nonpharmacological interventions are cheap and sometimes effective and should be considered for some patients.

If antihypertensive medication to control the blood pressure of the diabetic patient is needed, there are several interactions between the several types of antihypertensive drugs now commonly used and diabetes. Thiazides and thiazide-like diuretics produce deterioration of diabetic control and hyperglycaemia or overt diabetes mellitus in previously euglycaemic patients, most often the elderly (Lewis et al. 1976). The hyperglycaemia produced by the thiazides is thought to be related in part to the negative potassium balance produced by such drugs, although a direct effect on the insulin producing pancreatic beta cell has also been suggested. If thiazide-like drugs are used to treat diabetics, special attention must be paid to normalization of serum potassium. Since diabetic patients with nephropathy often have hyperkalaemia from hyporeninaemic hypoaldosteronism, diuretics such as spironolactone, triamterene or amiloride, which are potassium sparing, are best avoided in diabetic patients with renal insufficiency.

Antihypertensive drugs which have vasodilatory actions, such as hydralazine, may aggravate or expose latent coronary artery disease because of the attendant reflex sympathetic activation.

Antisympathetic agents such as guanethidine or reserpine may cause sympathetic dysfunction, including orthostatic hypotension and impotence in any patient. In the diabetic patient, who is already at risk for autonomic dysfunction from neuropathy, the threshold for such effects may be lower. The β-adrenergic blocking agents, now widely used to treat hypertension, need special consideration in the diabetic patient. Long-term diabetics develop a form of cardiomyopathy that may become symptomatic after β-blockade, with consequent congestive heart failure. Peripheral vascular disease from atherosclerosis may be produced or aggravated by nonspecific β-blockers given their capacity to block vasodilatory β_2-receptors in skeletal muscle arterioles. Insulin release can also be inhibited by β_2-blockade in type II diabetics, leading to deterioration of diabetic control. Nonspecific β-blockers carry special risks in the insulin-treated type I diabetic. First, glycogenolysis and gluconeogenesis also appear to be under β_2-mediation (Ostman 1983), and recovery from inadvertent hypoglycaemia may be impaired in diabetics with these counterregulatory mechanisms affected by nonspecific blockers. Also, the adrenaline response to hypoglycaemia is transformed into a pressor reaction with bradycardia in patients treated with nonselective blockers, and the sympathetic symptoms from hypoglycaemia might also be impaired. For all the above reasons, if one chooses a β-blocker in either a type I or type II diabetic, the cardioselective β_1-blockers are preferable.

Clonidine hydrochloride is another antihypertensive medication which affects sympathetic function. Several studies have reported that in high doses of clonidine impairs glucose tolerance in laboratory animals and in man (Metz et al. 1977). Given these potential effects, we sought to assess the effects of clonidine treatment on both glucose tolerance and diabetic control in patients with both hypertension and diabetes mellitus.

Patients and Methods

We studied 10 subjects with both mild hypertension (average diastolic blood pressures between 90 and 104 mmHg untreated) and type II diabetes mellitus, defined as two or more fasting serum glucose concentrations of greater than 140 mg/dl which was either previously untreated or was controlled by diet alone (seven patients), or an oral hypoglycaemic medication (three patients). Our patients ranged in age from 37 to 69 years, five were male and five were female, six were white and four were black. Eight were obese as defined by body weights above 120% of ideal. None had diabetic retinopathy or nephropathy.

Two weeks after cessation of all previous antihypertensive medications, we studied these patients by collecting a 24-hour urine specimen for electrolyte, aldosterone, and glucose excretion. After this collection and an overnight fast, patients rested supine for 45 minutes after which we drew blood samples for renin activity, aldosterone, catecholamines, glucose and glycohaemoglobin, and we then assessed sympathetic function in these patients by our standardised protocol using blood-pressure and pulse-rate responses to small graded doses of isoprenaline and phenylephrine to assess both adrenergic sensitivity and baroreflex function. One hour after adrenergic testing we injected 25 g of glucose i.v. for a glucose tolerance test and collected serial blood samples for glucose and insulin measurements over one hour.

We then treated these patients with clonidine 0.1 mg twice daily over the next ten weeks and instructed them to maintain their usual diets and standard activity, and specifically to neither gain nor lose weight. We measured weight, blood pressure, and fasting serum glucose weekly, and at the end of ten weeks, they re-collected 24-hour urine specimens and we re-performed sympathetic testing and the intravenous glucose tolerance test two hours after their last dose of clonidine.

Results

Clonidine treatment significantly reduced blood pressures in the supine, sitting, and standing postures in these patients and lowered average diastolic blood pressure to below 90 mmHg in all patients (Table 1). Side effects included dry mouth in five, drowsiness in two and partial erectile impotence in one. Plasma noradrenaline and adrenaline concentrations tended to be lower and sensitivity to exogenous isoprenaline was enhanced, although these changes were not significant. Clonidine increased the baroreflex slope in eight of ten patients and increased the mean slope significantly, but had no significant effects on renin activity or plasma or urinary aldosterone. Most relevantly, clonidine induced no significant changes in fasting serum glucose, urinary glucose excretion, or glycosylated haemoglobin concentration, although the former two tended to rise on the last measurements (Table 2). Mean body weight of our patients declined by 1.3 kg, but change in body weight did not correlate in any patient with changes in fasting glucose or other measurements of glucose sensitivity.

Table 1. Effects of Clonidine on Blood-pressure, Sympathetic and Baroreflex Function (mean + SE).

	Baseline	Clonidine
Supine blood pressure (mmHg)	146 ± 6/92 ± 3	129 ± 2/81 ± 1*
Sitting blood pressure	148 ± 5/93 ± 2	125 ± 4/80 ± 2*
Standing blood pressure	146 ± 6/94 ± 2	116 ± 4/77 ± 2*
Supine pulse	72 ± 4	68 ± 4
Plasma NA (pg/ml)	249 ± 1	181 ± 22
Plasma A (pg/ml)	25 ± 3	29 ± 7
CD-25 (μg isoprenaline)	2.6 ± 0.9	1.8 ± 0.4
PD-20 (μg phenylephrine)	59 ± 13	62 ± 20
Baroreflex slope (msec/mmHg)	5.5 ± 1.0	7.0 ± 1.2*

NA = Noradrenaline; A = Adrenaline; * $p < 0.05$

Table 2. Serum and Urinary Glucose and Glycohaemoglobin on Clonidine (mean + SE).

	1 (Baseline)	2	3	6	8	10
Weight (kg)	91.6 ± 5.1	91.9 ± 5.1	–	90.8 ± 4.9	90.7 ± 4.7	90.3 ± 4.3
Fasting glucose (mg/100 ml)	195 ± 18	195 ± 26	179 ± 14	179 ± 19	199 ± 25	231 ± 26
Urinary glucose (g)	27 ± 15	–	–	–	–	41 ± 16
Glycohaemo-globin (%)	10.1 ± 0.7	–	–	–	–	10.1 ± 0.9

The response to intravenous glucose yielded a greater incremental area under the glucose curve after clonidine treatment than before (Table 3), although no significant changes were seen under the insulin response curve. The K value for the disappearance rate of glucose was not significantly altered by clonidine.

Table 3. Effects of Clonidine on Intravenous Glucose Tolerance (mean + SE).

	Total Glucose AUC	Incremental Glucose AUC	Total Insulin AUC	Incremental Insulin AUC	K Value (%/min)
Baseline	468 ± 60	161 ± 13	401 ± 64	202 ± 49	0.59 ± 0.11
Clonidine	521 ± 53	184 ± 14*	410 ± 70	192 ± 61	0.52 ± 0.08

* $p < 0.05$, paired t-test.

Discussion

We thus found that treatment with clonidine of ten patients with both mild hypertension and type II diabetes mellitus for ten weeks produced blood pressure control in all and no significant changes in long term diabetic control as assessed by weekly fasting serum glucose, by glycosylated haemoglobin and by 24-hour urinary glucose excretions before and after treatment. We did, however, see minor alteration in glucose tolerance to intravenous glucose after clonidine treatment. Clonidine thus seems to be effective in these doses as monotherapy for the hypertension of diabetes.

For hypertensive diabetic patients, there appear to be some drugs that do not appreciably interact with diabetic control. Such drugs seem to include clonidine as mentioned, and prazosin, which does not produce reflex activation of the sympathetic nervous system (as occurs with other pure vasodilators). Although calcium channel antagonists have been reported to impair insulin release in high dosage, they appear not to adversely effect glucose tolerance in usual dosage, and might also be attractive agents. Since the hypertension of many diabetics seems to have accompanying sodium retention and extracellular fluid volume expansion, diuretics remain attractive drugs, and are effective. However, if they are used, effort should be made to normalize serum potassium, and to discontinue diuretic use if deterioration is seen of diabetic control. And, if one chooses to use a β-blocker, the β_1 cardioselective type seems to be preferable.

References

1. Christlieb AR (1973) Diabetes and hypertensive vascular disease. Am J Cardiol 32: 592–606
2. de Chatel R, Weidmann P, Flammer J, Ziegler WH, Beretta-Piccoli C, Vetter W, Reubi FC (1977) Sodium, renin, aldosterone, catecholamines, and blood pressure in diabetes mellitus. Kidney Int 12: 412–421
3. Hypertension Detection and Follow-up Program Cooperative Group (1979) Five year findings of the hypertension detection and follow-up program: reduction in mortality of persons with high blood pressure including mild hypertension. JAMA 242: 2562–2571
4. Knowler WC, Bennett PH, Ballintine EJ (1980) Increased incidence of retinopathy in diabetes with elevated blood pressure. N Engl J Med 302: 645–650
5. Krotkiewski M, Mandroukas K, Sjostrom L (1979) Effects of long-term physical training on body fat, metabolism and blood pressure in obesity. Metabolism 28: 650–658
6. Lewis PJ, Petrie A, Kohner EM, Dollery CT (1976) Deterioration of glucose tolerance in hypertension patients on prolonged diuretic treatment. Lancet 1: 564–566
7. MacGregor GA, Best FE, Cain JM (1982) Double-blinded randomised crossover trial of moderate sodium restriction in essential hypertension. Lancet 1: 351–354
8. Messerli FH (1982) Cardiovascular effects of obesity and hypertension. Lancet 1: 1163–1168
9. Metz SA, Halter JB, Robertson RP (1977) Induction of defective insulin secretion and impaired glucose tolerance by clonidine. Diabetes 27: 554–562
10. Mogenson CE (1982) Long-term antihypertensive treatment inhibiting progression of diabetic nephropathy. Br Med J 285: 685–688
11. Muichoodappa C, D'Elia JA, Libertino JA, Gleason RE, Christlieb AR (1979) Renal artery stenosis in hypertensive diabetics. J Urol 121: 555–558
12. Ostman J (1983) Beta-adrenergic blockade and diabetes mellitus – a review. Act Med Scand suppl 672: 69–77
13. Toth PJ, Horwitz RI (1983) Conflicting clinical trials and the uncertainty of treating mild hypertension. Am J Med 75: 482–487

Author's address:
Gordon P. Guthrie, Jr., M.D.
Department of Medicine
University of Kentucky
Lexington, Kentucky 40 536
U.S.A.

The Role of the Sympathetic Nervous System in the Control of Left Ventricular Mass in Hypertension

Jan I. M. Drayer and Michael A. Weber

Introduction

In the past, the electrocardiogram and the chest x-ray have been used in the diagnosis of left ventricular hypertrophy in patients with hypertension. The presence of signs of hypertrophy on the electrocardiogram or the presence of an enlarged heart on the chest x-ray were considered as an important prognostic marker of cardiovascular complications. In fact, data from the Framingham Study have revealed that the presence of cardiac hypertrophy is a more important risk factor than blood pressure itself (Kannel et al. 1970). The five year mortality rate increases with the presence of left ventricular hypertrophy from 7 to 38% in men and from 4 to 20% in women. The risk of clinical manifestations of cardiovascular disease also increases significantly with the presence of left ventricular hypertrophy on the electrocardiogram. Patients with hypertrophy more often had a myocardial infarction, angina, congestive heart failure, signs of occlusive peripheral vascular disease or cerebrovascular accidents than those without left ventricular hypertrophy (Kannel 1975). Successful antihypertensive therapy may lead to regression of signs of hypertrophy on the electrocardiogram (Freis 1980).

Unfortunately, cardiovascular disease occurs prior to the presence of abnormalities on the electrocardiogram in 78% of 35 to 44 year old men and in up to 45% of 55 to 64 year old men (Kannel 1979). Thus, the electrocardiogram is not a very specific prognostic tool in the evaluation of hypertensive patients. Recently, the echocardiogram has been used in the diagnosis of left ventricular hypertrophy in hypertension. Echocardiographic left ventricular hypertrophy was found in 48% of hypertensive patients. The incidence of left ventricular hypertrophy detected using the electrocardiogram or the chest x-ray was less than 5% in the same patient population (Savage et al. 1979). It has become evident that the echocardiogram provides a more specific and sensitive tool in the diagnosis of left ventricular hypertrophy than the electrocardiogram or the chest x-ray.

Blood pressure itself is the most important aetiological factor in the development of cardiac hypertrophy. Blood pressure and, more specifically, systolic blood pressure, is the main determinant of cardiac work load on left ventricular wall stress. A direct correlation between systolic blood pressure and left ventricular mass has been found in many studies. In addition, cardiac muscle mass tends to regress during successful antihypertensive therapy (Drayer et al. 1984). However, recent studies in animals and in man have shown that it is unlikely that blood pressure is the only aetiological factor in the development of left

Hypertension Center, Veterans Administration Medical Center, Long Beach, California, and the University of California, Irvine, California, U.S.A.

ventricular hypertrophy in hypertensive patients. It has been shown that signs of hypertrophy may be present in patients before the development of high blood pressure. Moreover, cardiac hypertrophy often is found in patients with mild hypertension and in adolescents with hypertension. In addition, it has been shown that control of hypertension does not necessarily lead to decreases in left ventricular mass or to regression of cardiac hypertrophy (for review see Drayer et al. 1984; Drayer et al. 1983a).

Left Ventricular Hypertrophy: Experiments in Animals

Studies using myocardial cells from rats have shown that noradrenaline can produce hypertrophy of myocytes through stimulation of α-receptors and that the effects of noradrenaline on cell growth can be blocked using the α-adrenergic antagonist, prazosin, but not after blockade of β-receptors with propranolol. Addition of noradrenaline to the tissue bath resulted in a 50% increase in myocyte volume which was completely blocked when prazosin or phentolamine was present in the tissue bath (Simpson 1983).
Ruskoaha (1983) has shown that the development of cardiac hypertrophy in spontaneously hypertensive rats can be prevented by administration of prazosin. The ventricular weight/body weight ratio was 3.6 ± 0.05 mg/g in control animals and 3.4 ± 0.03 mg/g in rats treated with prazosin 0.0625 mg/ml in drinking water ($p < 0.02$). This observation does not exclude a role of blood pressure in the determination of cardiac muscle mass, since prazosin lowered blood pressure significantly from 184 ± 2 mmHg in control animals to 166 ± 3 mmHg in treated rats. However, other drugs tested, such as the vasodilator, minoxidil, actually caused an increase in left ventricular mass (3.6 ± 0.05 in control animals and 3.9 ± 0.05 mg/g in minoxidil treated rats, $p < 0.001$) despite control of blood pressure (184 ± 2 in untreated and 169 ± 3 mmHg in treated rats). Sen (1983) and Pegram and Frohlich (1983) had shown previously that hydralazine therapy fails to cause regression of cardiac muscle mass. In contrast, drugs which block the sympathetic nervous system successfully reduced cardiac muscle mass in spontaneously hypertensive rats. α-methyldopa caused a reduction in cardiac mass from 3.5 ± 0.06 to 2.8 ± 0.05 mg/g ($p < 0.01$). In the study by Pegram and Frohlich (1983), heart weight decreased from 2.2 to 1.9 mg/g ($p < 0.05$) during therapy with clonidine and from 3.5 to 3.3 mg/g ($p < 0.05$) during therapy with α-methyldopa. These data suggest that, at least in animal experiments, the sympathetic nervous system plays an important role in the development of cardiac hypertrophy. The role of the β-adrenergic receptor in this regard has not been clearly elucidated. According to the studies by Simpson et al. (1983), β-adrenergic receptors are not involved in the regulation of the increase in the volume of myocytes induced by noradrenaline. However, in these experiments, the beating of the heart cells (workload) was affected by the β-adrenergic antagonist, propranolol. Sen (1983) has shown that propranolol did not significantly alter cardiac mass in spontaneously hypertensive rats; heart weight was 3.5 ± 0.06 mg/g in control animals and 3.2 ± 0.04 mg/g (NS) in propranolol treated animals. In contrast, Ruskoaha (1983) has shown that metoprolol successfully ($p < 0.02$) reduced cardiac mass in these rats; from 3.4 ± 0.03 to 3.2 ± 0.05 mg/g. In fact, he has shown that combined blockade of α- and β-adrenergic receptors was slightly more effective in decreasing muscle mass than monotherapy with prazosin or metoprolol. Heart weight was 3.3 ± 0.03 in animals treated with the α- and β-adrenergic antagonist, labetalol, and 3.6 ± 0.07 in control rats

(p < 0.01). It is conceivable that the regression of hypertrophy observed during therapy with the combined α- and β-adrenergic antagonist is related to the drug-induced decrease in sympathetic nervous system activity, decreased cardiac workload as well as the fall in blood pressure.

These observations in animal experiments can be summarized as follows. Stimulation of α- and/or β-adrenergic receptors plays a role in the development of cardiac hypertrophy in the spontaneously hypertensive rat. The sympathetic nervous system clearly is involved in this process. Regression of hypertrophy may occur during antihypertensive therapy, but only when the blood pressure is controlled using sympatholytic agents. Agents which lower blood pressure but at the same stimulate the sympathetic nervous system (e.g. vasodilators such as hydralazine or minoxidil) fail to cause regression of cardiac muscle mass. In addition, these drugs do not prevent the development of cardiac hypertrophy in spontaneously hypertensive rats. Sympatholytic agents are so effective in causing a reduction in cardiac mass that they do so even in the absence of control blood pressure (Tomanek et al. 1982; Kuwajima et al. 1982). This finding is in agreement with the observation that subpressor doses of noradrenaline can cause cardiac hypertrophy (Garner and Laks 1980).

Left Ventricular Hypertrophy: Relationship to Cardiac Function

It has been shown that the presence of cardiac hypertrophy is related to a dramatic increase in cardiovascular complications in man. The presence of left ventricular hypertrophy also causes significant changes in cardiac function. Systolic function often is reduced in patients with hypertrophy (Inouye et al. 1984). These diastolic function abnormalities might be an early indicator of the development of hypertrophy.

The relationship between cardiac function and hypertrophy has been further studied. Ayobe and Tarazi (1983) have shown that hypertrophy leads to a decrease in the density of β-adrenergic receptors. They claim that the decrease in inotropic responsiveness to β-stimulation ultimately is responsible for the left ventricular failure of the hypertrophied heart. Coronary vascular reserve also becomes progressively impaired in the hypertrophied heart, which has a low work efficiency and an increased oxygen consumption. Obviously, the progression from hypertrophy to heart failure will be significantly affected by the co-presence of coronary artery disease. Borkon et al. (1982) has shown that animals with infracoronary obstruction and cardiac hypertrophy have a greater susceptibility to the development of subendocardial ischemia than animals without hypertrophy. In addition Wicker et al. (1982) showed that a decrease in blood pressure in the hypertrophied heart does adversely affect coronary flow reserve.

Thus to preserve cardiac function a reduction in blood pressure should coincide with regression of cardiac hypertrophy. Capaso et al. (1982) demonstrated that reduction of blood pressure together with regression of hypertrophy will not adversely affect cardiac function.

The data from the animal experiments suggest that in the course of the development of hypertension both blood pressure and the sympathetic nervous system will alter cardiac muscle mass. Initially, a moderate degree of hypertrophy will not cause a significant decrease in cardiac function. However, more severe forms of hypertrophy or the presence of coronary artery disease will induce significant decreases in diastolic and systolic function of the heart. Treatment of the hypertension should not only focus on the control of blood pressure but it should also take into account the effects of therapy on the heart. Sympatholytic agents seem to lower blood pressure effectively and, at the same time, they have a beneficial effect on cardiac mass. Control of both blood pressure and cardiac mass does not seem to have a deleterious effect on cardiac function.

Left Ventricular Hypertrophy: Human Data

Recent publications have revealed that regression of cardiac muscle mass may occur in the course of antihypertensive therapy in man (for review see Drayer et al. 1984; Drayer et al. 1983a). The data published confirm the results of the animal studies described earlier.

The analysis of the data available in man shows that baseline muscle mass, blood pressure, and the activity of the sympathetic nervous system are the main factors which determine the degree of regression of cardiac mass during antihypertensive therapy. Patients who had significant left ventricular hypertrophy prior to the start of therapy will show regression of muscle mass more readily than patients without clear hypertrophy (Drayer et al. 1984). Blood pressure control seems to be a less important factor in the regression of muscle mass. The correlation between changes in blood pressure and changes in cardiac mass are weak or not significant in most studies. Moreover, we have shown recently that the fall in pressure observed in patients who experienced regression of cardiac mass was not greater than the fall observed in patients in whom muscle mass did not decrease during antihypertensive treatment. However, when all data published are taken together, a significant relationship between blood pressure control and changes in cardiac mass was observed: $r = 0.83$, $p < 0.001$ (Drayer et al. 1983a). Additional information supporting the role of blood pressure in the development and regression of left ventricular hypertrophy is represented in the close relationship between results of long-term blood pressure monitoring and echocardiographic left ventricular mass. The correlation coefficient between the average of systolic blood pressure measured during a whole-day and left ventricular mass is highly significant: $r = 0.81$, $p < 0.01$ (Drayer et al. 1983c). These correlations are much stronger than those observed between casual blood pressures and left ventricular mass. Thus, careful evaluation of blood pressure and cardiac mass does reveal a fairly close relationship between the two parameters. However, this relationship does not exclude a role for other factors such as the sympathetic nervous system in the development of cardiac hypertrophy in hypertensive patients.

We have reported that regression of muscle mass was not observed during therapy with a diuretic, a vasodilator or the combination of both drugs (Drayer et al. 1982; Drayer et al 1983b). Hydrochlorothiazide therapy resulted in a significant decrease in blood pressure from $155 \pm 3/104 \pm 2$ to $144 \pm 3/98 \pm 2$ mmHg (n = 20, $p < 0.01$). However, left ventricular muscle mass did not change significantly (from 238 ± 11 to 224 ± 10 g, NS). Similar findings have been reported by Wollam et al. (1983). Treatment with the vasodilator trimazosin resulted in a decrease in blood pressure from $154 \pm 6/100 \pm 1$ to $141 \pm 4/90 \pm 2$ mmHg (n = 11, $p < 0.05$) but left ventricular mass did not change significantly (from 268 ± 20 to 253 ± 18 g, NS). Therapy with a combination of a diuretic and a vasodilator lowered blood pressure markedly (from $152 \pm 6/102 \pm 3$ to $134 \pm 6/92 \pm 3$ mmHg; n = 9; $p < 0.001$) but again a significant change in muscle mass was not observed (from 234 ± 16 to 242 ± 15 g, NS). Preliminary results of antihypertensive therapy with the calcium channel blocker, nitrendipine, indicate that this vasodilator does not lead to a significant change in muscle mass, despite its potent hypotensive action.

It seems evident that control of blood pressure is not the only factor in the regulation of cardiac mass. Apparently, treatment with drugs that lower blood pressure but, at the same time, stimulate the activity of the sympathetic nervous system will not lead to regression of cardiac mass. Similarly, regression of cardiac mass was not observed during therapy with β-blockers that have intrinsic sympathomimetic activity. In fact, cardiac muscle mass increased slightly during therapy with pindolol (from 210 ± 37 to 240 ± 37 g, NS) and during therapy with acebutolol: from 233 ± 13 to 246 ± 17 g (Plotnick et al. 1984; Drayer et al. 1984). In another study, it was shown that regression of cardiac muscle mass was not observed in patients in whom acebutolol failed to decrease heart rate, or failed to reduce sympathetic nervous system activity (Trimarco et al. 1984).

In contrast to these rather disappointing findings, it has been shown that antihypertensive therapy with a sympatholytic action successfully reduced cardiac mass. Treatment with β-adrenergic antagonists which do not possess intrinsic sympathomimetic activity have shown to cause regression of left ventricular mass. It is possible that this decrease in muscle mass is related to the decrease in blood pressure induced by these agents as well as to specific pharmacologic properties of these drugs. β-adrenergic antagonists decrease cardiac output, cardiac workload and cardiac oxygen consumption. Moreover, the drugs decrease the output of noradrenaline at the nerve terminal. Regression of hypertrophy has been observed during treatment with atenolol, metoprolol, nadolol, propranolol and timolol (for review see Drayer et al. 1983a).

We have shown that therapy with centrally-acting sympatholytic agents such as α-methyldopa results in a significant decrease in cardiac muscle mass (Drayer et al. 1983d). In this study, 12 patients with diuretic resistant hypertension were treated with α-methyldopa. Prior to the start of therapy, septal and or posterior wall thickness exceeded 11 mm in seven of these patients. At the end of the study, all patients had a septal and posterior wall thickness of less than 11 mm. These data have been confirmed by others. Wollam et al. (1983) reported a significant decrease in cardiac muscle mass during therapy with α-methyldopa with, or without, hydrochlorothiazide. They reported that septal thickness did not decrease in any of the patients treated with a diuretic alone. In contrast, septal thickness decreased in 16 of the 20 patients treated with α-methyldopa with, or without, a diuretic. Corea et al. (1981) have shown that left ventricular mass index decreased from 87 ± 3 to 77 ± 3 g/m^2, p < 0.01, in patients treated with this centrally-acting sympatholytic agent. Finally, Fouad et al. (1982) have reported that, during therapy with α-methyldopa, regression of cardiac muscle mass may occur even in the absence of control of blood pressure. Thus, decreases in left ventricular muscle mass are frequently observed during therapy with antihypertensive agents which inhibit sympathetic nervous system activity. Apparently, additional therapy with a low dose of a diuretic does not affect the outcome of sympatholytic agents on left ventricular mass (Drayer et al. 1983a). Actually, addition of the diuretic might enhance the beneficial effect of sympatholytic agents on cardiac mass. It will be shown, in a study by McMahon et al., in the next chapter of this book, that regression of cardiac hypertrophy also is observed in patients treated with the centrally-acting sympatholytic agent, clonidine. In this study, a highly significant decrease in left ventricular mass was observed.

Finally, new drug delivery systems may further help control left ventricular mass in hypertensive patients. Transdermal therapy with clonidine results in control of blood pressure continuously during the day. It is conceivable that continuous release of small amounts of this drug will provide a smoother control of blood pressure over the day than oral therapy. Thus, average whole-day blood pressure will be decreased further and, in view of the close relationship between whole-day blood pressure average and left ventricular mass, the latter might show an even more marked regression during antihypertensive therapy with transdermal clonidine.

References

1. Ayobe MH, Tarazi RC (1983) β-receptors and contractile reserve in left ventricular hypertrophy. Hypertension 5: I191–I197
2. Borken AM, Jones M, Bell JH, Pierce JE (1982) Regional myocardial blood flow in left ventricular hypertrophy. J Thorac Cardiovasc Surg 84: 876–885
3. Capasso JM, Strobeck JE, Malhotra A, Scheuer J, Sonnenblick EH (1982) Contractile behavior of rat myocardium after reversal of hypertensive hypertrophy. Am J Physiol 242: H882–H889
4. Corea L, Bentivoglio M, Verdecchia P (1981) Reversal of left ventricular hypertrophy in essential hypertension by early and long-term treatment with methyldopa. Clin Trials J 18: 380–394
5. Drayer JIM, Gardin JM, Weber MA, Aronow WS (1982) Changes in ventricular septal thickness during diuretic therapy. Clin Pharmacol Ther 32: 283–288
6. Drayer JIM, Gardin JM, Weber MA (1983a) Echocardiographic left ventricular hypertrophy in hypertension. Chest 84: 217–221
7. Drayer JIM, Gardin JM, Weber MA (1983b) Changes in cardiac muscle mass during vasodilation therapy of hypertension. Clin Pharmacol Ther 33: 727–732
8. Drayer JIM, Weber MA, DeYoung JL (1983c) Blood pressure as a determinant of cardiac left ventricular muscle mass. Arch Intern Med 143: 90–92
9. Drayer JIM, Weber MA, Gardin JM, Lipson JL (1983d) The effect on long-term antihypertensive therapy on cardiac anatomy in patients with essential hypertension. Am J Med 75: 116–120
10. Drayer JIM, Weber MA, Gardin JM (1984) Cardiac left ventricular muscle mass and end-systolic wall stress during antihypertensive therapy. In: Messerli F and Tarazi RC (eds) The Heart and Hypertension. In press
11. Fouad FM, Nakashima Y, Tarazi RC, Salcedo EE (1982) Reversal of left ventricular hypertrophy in hypertensive patients treated with methyldopa. Am J Cardiol 49: 795–801
12. Freis ED (1980) Electrocardiographic changes in the course of antihypertensive treatment. Am J Med 75: 111–115
13. Garner, D, Laks M (1980) Is the physiological hypertrophy produced by a 3 month subhypertensive norepinephrine infusion blocked by propranolol? Circulation 62 (Suppl 3): 68
14. Inouye I, Massie B, Loge D, Tonic N, Silverstein D, Simpson P, Tubau J (1984) Abnormal left ventricular filling: An early finding in mild to moderate systemic hypertension. Am J Cardiol 53: 120–126
15. Kannel WB, Gordon T, Castelli WP, Margolis JR (1970) Electrographic left ventricular hypertrophy and risk of coronary heart disease. The Framingham Study. Ann Int Med 72: 813–822
16. Kannel WB (1975) Epidemiology and Control of Hypertension. Paul O (ed) Yearbook Medical Publications, Chicago, p. 553–598
17. Kannel WB (1979) Theories and Use of β-blockers in Hypertension and Angina. Roberts RH (ed) Yearbook Medical Publications, Chicago
18. Kuwajima I, Kardon MB, Pegram BL, Sesoko S, Frohlich ED (1982) Regression of left ventricular hypertrophy in two-kidney one-clip Goldblatt hypertension. Hypertension 4: 113–118
19. Pegram BL, Frohlich ED (1983) Cardiovascular adjustment to antiadrenergic agents. Am J Med 75: 94–99
20. Plotnick GD, Fisher ML, Wohl B, Hamilton JH, Hamilton BP (1984) Improvement in depressed cardiac function in hypertensive patients during pindolol treatment. Am J Med 76: 25–30

21. Ruskoaha H (1983) Effects of drug treatment on hypertension and cardiac hypertrophy in spontaneously hypertensive rats. Acta Univ Ouluensis, D96, Pharmacol Physiol 17
22. Savage DD, Drayer JIM, Henry WL, Mathews EC Jr, Ware JH, Gardin JM (1979) Echocardiographic assessment of cardiac anatomy and function in hypertensive subjects. Circulation 59: 623–632
23. Sen S (1983) Regression of cardiac hypertrophy. Experimental animal model. Am J Med 75: 87–93
24. Simpson P (1983) Norepinephrine-stimulated hypertrophy of cultured rat myocardial cells is an alpha-I adrenergic response. J Clin Invest 72: 732–738
25. Tomanek RJ, Bhatnagar RK, Schmid P, Brody MJ (1982) Role of catecholamines in myocardial cell hypertrophy in hypertensive rats. Am J Physiol 242: H1015–1021
26. Trimarco B, Ricciardelli B, DeLuca N, Volpe M, Veniero A, Cuocolo A, Condorelli M (1984) Effect of acebutolol on left ventricular hemodynamics and anatomy in systemic hypertension. Am J Cardiol 53: 791–796
27. Wicker P, Tarawi R, Dallocchio M, Bricard H (1982) Coronary flow in experimental cardiac hypertrophy caused by arterial hypertension. Arch Mal Coeur 75: 133–136
28. Wollam GL, Hall WD, Porter VD, Douglas MB, Unger DJ, Blumenstein BA, Cotsonis GA, Knudtson ML, Felner JM, Schlant RC (1983) Time course of regression of left ventricular hypertrophy in treated hypertensive patients. Am J Med 75: 100–110

Authors' address:
Jan I. M. Drayer, M.D.
Hypertension Center
Veterans Administration Medical Center
5901 East Seventh Street
Long Beach, California 90822
U.S.A.

Discussion

MATHIAS:

The sympathetic nervous system, especially noradrenaline, causes lipolysis and will increase plasma concentrations of the free fatty acids. Is it known whether clonidine, because of its marked sympatholytic effect, can impair lipolysis and perhaps have some clinically significant impact on the plasma lipids?

DIEHM:

There are some preliminary data suggesting that the centrally-acting antihypertensive agents may produce decreases in plasma cholesterol concentrations, but as yet there have been no major prospective studies to evaluate the overall lipid effects.

MEYERS:

Several years ago we reported that D-propranolol had an effect on glucose tolerance, and actually appeared to cause an increase in blood glucose concentration. D-propranolol, as you know, possesses no β-blocking activity, although like DL-propranolol it does exhibit marked local anaesthetic activity. Is it known whether this property might explain the actions of propranolol on glucose and insulin, and could it have been a factor in the studies presented by Dr. Guthrie?

GUTHRIE:

It is difficult to be certain as to the clinical importance of the local anaesthetic properties of propranolol. Most studies comparing D- and DL-propranolol have used fairly high doses, and it is not really certain how relevant the local anaesthetic characteristics of the drug might be in the usual clinical setting. The effect on glucose tolerance I reported with propranolol has also been observed with other non-selective β-blockers such as timolol. Other investigators have compared propranolol with metoprolol in their effects on glucose, and have shown that the fasting glucose concentration during propranolol was significantly increased during treatment, whereas values during metoprolol treatment remained unchanged. Hence, I believe that the evidence indicates that the effect on glucose tolerance is mediated through the actions of the non-selective β-blockers at their receptors rather than through local anaesthetic properties.

HOUSTON:

It would appear from the recent literature, particularly the Framingham data and also the Lipid Research Centers trial, that small changes in total cholesterol can produce significant reductions in coronary heart disease. Moreover, certain ratios of the lipids have some strong predictive properties, particulary the total cholesterol to HDL ratio. The HDL_2 subfraction is probably the most important component of HDL in predicting coronary disease. Although the changes in lipids during Dr. Diehm's study were relatively small, and usually not significant, I still wonder whether over a long treatment period of 30 to 40 years they might have an impact on the likelihood of coronary disease, and whether we should take this into account when considering drugs for the treatment of hypertension.

DIEHM:

At this stage it is obviously not possible for me to provide definitive data in this area, but I think your speculation is really very interesting. Clearly, long-term studies are required.

FRANKLIN:

I think it is important, as Dr. Diehm has suggested, to consider long-term studies. I think we might have been misled by relatively short-term studies of diuretic treatment of hypertension in which it appeared that lipid abnormalities were being produced. However, in the long-term Hypertension Detection and Follow-up study, in which there were some disturbances in lipid metabolism initially, follow-up data after 12 months of treatment indicated that lipid values had returned to normal. There is also a question of dosage, especially with diuretics. We are now entering a period in which we are concerned about the consequences of excessive doses of diuretics, and it is quite possible that as we start using smaller diuretic doses some of these metabolic problems will become less com mon and less severe.

MATHIAS:

I think we have been impressed with the potential simplicity and attractiveness of using the transdermal clonidine as single-agent therapy, but I wonder how well patients would respond if they were taking this preparation as part of a multiple-dose regimen. For example, how do patients react to using the transdermal clonidine, applied on a once-weekly basis, in combination with diuretics being administered on a once-daily basis?

DRAYER:

There has been a change during the last few years in the way we are using antihypertensive agents. We are now much more aware of the biochemical and physical side-effects of treatment, and much of our modern strategy is devoted to minimizing these problems. Obviously, the use of low doses is a key component of this approach. Thus, I believe the chief attribute of transdermal clonidine to be its ability to produce only minimal side-effects, and I would have no hesitation in using it in combination with oral medications if I felt that this mixed approach would provide therapeutic efficacy while at the same time avoiding adverse effects. Preliminary reports from investigators who have administered the transdermal clonidine in patients simultaneously taking once-daily diuretics indicate that these patients are very satisfied with this form of combination treatment.

KELLAWAY:

In the glucose data presented by Dr. Guthrie there appeared to be an increase in urinary excretion of glucose towards the end of the clonidine treatment period. Was this significant?

GUTHRIE:

There was an apparent trend towards an increase in urinary glucose measurements at the end of the study, but this was not significant. There was some fluctuation in this measurement during the study, and this might help explain the appearance of that trend. The fact that glycohaemoglobin did not change during the 10 weeks of the study seems to indicate that the clonidine treatment did not produce any notable changes in glucose metabolism.

WHEATHLEY:

I agree with Dr. Guthrie's assessment, but there did seem to be a tendency for plasma glucose concentrations to increase during the study. If the observation had been carried out over a longer period, perhaps six or 12 months, do you think that we might have seen a significant increase in blood glucose concentrations or is that purely speculative at this point?

GUTHRIE:

There is some theoretical basis to suspect that clonidine and related drugs might influence glucose tolerance. Studies with pure α-agonists performed in animal models have indicated that there might be some impairment of insulin release. There does not appear to be any systematic data in humans. In the studies we have presented here we saw a change only on one occasion, albeit at the end of the study I cannot say whether a longer period of observation would have allowed a more marked trend to develop, but studies with this class of drugs in diabetic hypertensive patients have not revealed any clear-cut changes in glucose levels or in treatment requirements for diabetes.

BOEKHORST:

The β-blocking drugs have been shown to have an adverse effect on plasma lipid concentrations. Total cholesterol concentrations may increase, whereas the concentration of the HDL fraction may go down. There might also be adverse effects on triglycerides. In patients with underlying ischaemic heart disease, and who have a tendency to lipid abnormalities, would it be prudent to prescribe β-blockers? Should we consider the concurrent use of lipid-lowering strategies in such patients if β-blockers are given?

DIEHM:

These are interesting theoretical concerns, and clearly more work is required. To the best of my knowledge, however, we do not have any clear-cut clinical data indicating that β-blockers exhibit adverse effects under these circumstances.

DRAYER:

Drugs such as the β-blockers have several actions, some of which are beneficial and others, as we have already discussed, which might be adverse. Thus, even though we might be concerned about deleterious changes in the lipid profile during β-blockers treatment, these could be more than adequately compensated for by the concurrent decrease in blood pressure, reduction in oxygen requirements of the myocardium, and even the antiarrhythmic properties of this class of drug. I believe that the secondary prevention trials with the β-blockers, which have indicated that they decrease death rates in patients who have had a myocardial infarction, suggest that these agents provide a clear-cut benefit. Of course, it would be most interesting to see secondary or even primary prevention trials carried out with drugs which do not have a potential for adverse lipid changes. Perhaps we might then see some even stronger benefits. The same argument could also be made for diuretics. Even though they are very useful for the treatment of hypertension, it is possible that their effects on lipids and their other metabolic effects prevent the full expression of the potential reduction in major cardiovascular complications.

SOWERS:

One of the characteristics of hypertension in diabetes is an expanded plasma volume and an increase in total exchangeable sodium. I should like to know whether Dr. Guthrie evaluated the effect of clonidine treatment on either of these parameters in his diabetic patients who were treated for hypertension.

GUTHRIE:

We believe that the sodium space is about 10% higher in diabetic hypertensives than it is in non-diabetic hypertensive patients. For that reason, many investigators have advocated the use of diuretics in the treatment of hypertension in diabetics, and have found these drugs to be effective. We do not yet know what effect clonidine has on the sodium space. In fact, the effects of clonidine on sodium metabolism in general are controversial. Some studies have indicated that clonidine actually produces a net loss of sodium, whereas others have found no change or even some retention.

WEBER:

There have been some interesting studies recently by Campese dealing with these questions in elderly patients, although I do not think that he included individuals with diabetes. During six weeks of single-agent therapy with clonidine in a fairly large group of older patients with hypertension, he noted significant decreases in both plasma volume and total exchangeable sodium. These changes were also associated with decreases in plasma noradrenaline concentrations and a marked fall in blood pressure.

SAMBHI:

During treatment with the transdermal clonidine preparation, is there a relationship between the number or size of the patches administered and the plasma concentration that is achieved?

DRAYER:

We were quite impressed with the consistency of the plasma clonidine concentrations, especially during treatment with the single small patch. They averaged around 0.3 ng/ml, and almost all observations fell within the range 0.15 to 0.45 ng/ml. In our experience, when we used more than one patch the plasma clonidine concentrations were higher, although there did seem to be some variability. On the other hand, some of the early pharmacokinetic studies performed by Shaw and her co-workers indicated a very tight relationship between the size or number of transdermal patches used and the ensuing concentration of clonidine in the plasma.

BOEKHORST:

We know that diuretics can have an adverse effect on glucose tolerance, and may make the treatment of diabetes more difficult, but there are many diabetic patients with hypertension who require diuretic treatment for effective control of their blood pressure. Is it still correct to say that frusemide is preferable to the thiazide diuretics in such patients?

GUTHRIE:

I would agree that the thiazide group of diuretics is probably the least preferable in this setting, perhaps because they can induce hypokalaemia and also because of their effects on serum lipids. Frusemide can work well in these patients, and may be less likely to have a suppressive effect on endogenous insulin secretion. Another possibility is the newer diuretic, indapamide; some studies have indicated that this agent produces fewer metabolic side-effects than lany other presently available diuretics.

54

Clonidine Transdermal Delivery System: Cutaneous Toxicity Studies

Howard Maibach

Introduction

In February 1983, European investigators conducting clinical trials to evaluate the efficacy of the clonidine transdermal device (Catapres-TTS) reported the first cases of dermatitis severe enough to necessitate discontinuation of therapy (Boekhorst 1983; Groth et al. 1983). The manifestations of this dermatitic reaction were pruritis, erythema and, less frequently, vesiculation of the skin beneath the transdermal patch. Depending on the geographical location of the centre reporting, as well as the size of the population being tested, the incidence of skin reactions varied between five and 30%. Some of the patients with moderate to severe skin signs seemingly demonstrated sensitization to some component of the clonidine device.

Although a few subjects developed reactions following only five days of transdermal treatment, analysis of preliminary data indicated that 90% of the dermatitic reactions presumptively diagnosed as allergic contact dermatitis occurred later on during the first

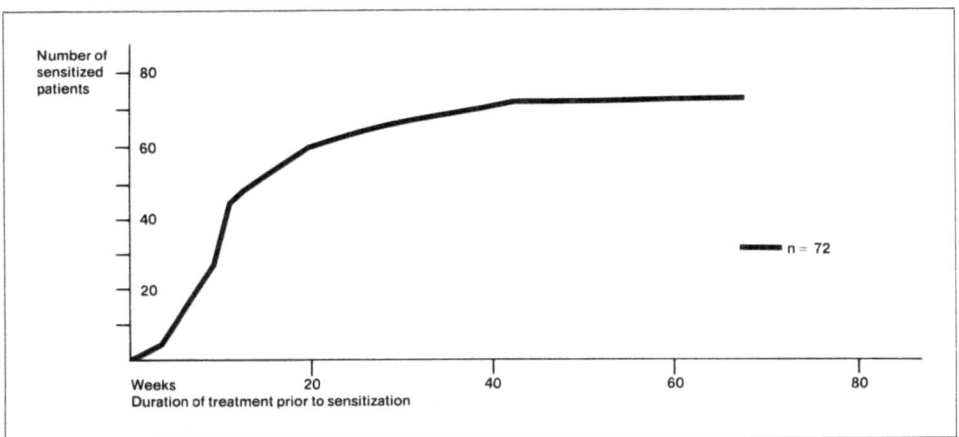

Fig. 1. Relationship of treatment duration to development of cantact sensitization in 72 sensitized patients.

Department of Dermatology, University of California, School of Medicine, Moffitt Hospital, San Francisco U.S.A., and Harley Street, London, U.K.

twenty weeks of therapy (Fig. 1). Therapeutic duration is an important factor in the sensitization process. Since an allergic response requires a week to many weeks to develop, it seemed possible that these patients were manifesting Type IV delayed hypersensitivity reactions resulting in allergic contact dermatitis.

To determine the long-term safety of the clonidine transdermal device, the quantitative incidence of allergic contact dermatitis had to be established, and the qualitative nature of the reaction and its potential consequences clarified. Thus, patients in Switzerland and Holland suspected of allergic dermatitis subsequent to contact sensitization received diagnostic patch testing. Investigators utilized a variety of test materials to isolate which of the individual components of the clonidine device was the responsible sensitizing agent (Maibach 1984). This investigation followed the recommendations of the International Contact Dermatitis Research Group (ICDRG), placing the test materials in Finn chambers and occluding the skin over a 24–48 hour period. Based on ICDRG grading criteria (Wilkinson et al. 1970), the results confirmed seven of the eight cases as delayed-type sensitization, the patients reacting to clonidine-containing material only (Boekhorst 1983; Groth et al. 1983; Maibach 1984). Repeat patch testing on a second group of possibly sensitized patients utilizing clonidine components that included LUE, a molecule formed by a clonidine-acetaldehyde reaction, again elicited skin signs confirming Type IV hypersensitivity.

As a result of these patient studies proving contact sensitization, we reviewed the previously performed dermatotoxicity testing of this product to determine why the investigations failed to predict the observed contact sensitization. Noting that the sample size of prior work may have been too small to be predictive, we suspected that additional dermatotoxicity testing might assist in delineating factors contributing to sensitization while pinpointing the chemical nature of the sensitizer. Although patch testing demonstrated that clonidine in petrolatum could elicit a reaction in sensitized patients, this form of enquiry would not distinguish among a) clonidine, b) a preparation impurity, c) a clonidine metabolite or d) clonidine combined with or reacting to a component of the device as the specific sensitizing agent.

We designed a protocol to, first, clarify whether clonidine alone or in combination with a device component was the most likely sensitizer, while, secondly, increasing the population sample size to a more statistically relevant level to better quantify true incidence.

Methods

Our first study repeated the 21-day cumulative irritancy assay on a group of 28 Caucasian male and female volunteers ranging in age from 18 to 60 years. To a 1.0 cm² epidermal site on the upper back, each subject received applications of the following test materials. 1) 3% clonidine in petrolatum and 2) petrolatum as a control were applied in Finn chambers with plastic occlusive (Blenderm) tape, while 3) the clonidine device (Catapres-TTS) and 4) the transdermal placebo device were self-adhesive. For 5 days, each item remained in place for 24 hours, followed by daily removal and inspection and grading of the site for evidence of reaction before reapplication. On the fifth day, each applied item remained in place over the weekend. This procedure was repeated for a total of 21 days. Analysis of the results indicated that the clonidine device caused a greater reaction than 3% clonidine in petrolatum, averaging scores of 1.2 and 0.4 respectively. The highest

56

score with the clonidine device was 6.5, cumulative over 21 days, while with 3% clonidine in petrolatum it was 3.5 after 21 days. The average score represents the total score divided by the number of subjects. However, comparing the results to the values of the scoring scale shows the clonidine device to be only a mild irritant (Table 1).

Table 1. Scoring Scale Employed for Evaluating Skin Reactions.

0	= Negative
+–	= Equivocal reaction
1	= Erythema
2	= Erythema and induration
3	= Erythema, induration and vesicles
4	= Erythema, induration and bullae

These same subjects next underwent a delayed challenge for allergic contact sensitization to the test materials following 10 days of no exposure. After 48 hour application to a lateral arm site, evaluation for sensitization was performed one hour post removal (49 hours) and at 96 hours, two days later. All sites proved negative.

A second 21-day cumulative irritancy assay performed on a similar group of 28 volunteers utilized the following test materials on a 1.0 cm² skin site: 1) 1% clonidine in petrolatum, 2) 3% clonidine in petrolatum, 3) 9% clonidine in petrolatum, 4) 3% clonidine and 0.03% LU 92 in petrolatum, and 5) petrolatum, as a control. As with the previous investigation, the materials were applied in Finn chambers, attached to the skin with plastic occlusive tape for 24 hours, then removed to allow evaluation of skin reaction before reapplication of fresh test materials. Applications done on the fifth day remained in place over the weekend.

At the conclusion of this study, no significant difference in skin reaction among the sites receiving clonidine in petrolatum at varying strengths could be perceived; scores (Table 1) averaged 0.9, 1.2, 1.0 and 1.0 respectively. Again, clonidine in petrolatum proved to be a modest skin irritant comparable to certain commercially-prepared lubricating lotions. However, delayed challenge did not demonstrate evidence of contact sensitization.

The third investigation, a modified Draize skin sensitization study, was performed on two separate groups of 105 and 93 healthy male and female volunteers ranging in age from 18 to 67 years. Group I received three weekly applications of 9% clonidine in petrolatum, and petrolatum as a control, to a specific, repeated skin site. Each application was left in place for seven days. Group II underwent a similar procedure utilizing the clonidine device and a transdermal placebo device as a control. After 21 days, all of the volunteers in both groups received a 72 hour challenge at a fresh skin site.

Following the first challenge, two additional successive weekly applications were reinstituted at the previously used skin site. Each group received induction with the same testing materials used prior to the challenge. At the end of 14 days, we performed a 48 hour challenge. Both the first and second challenges utilized the same test materials as the induction, but different skin sites. These were evaluated just after removal of the challenge, and at 24 or 48 hours post removal.

Group I, induced with 9% clonidine in petrolatum, had essentially negative scores following both challenges. However, Group II manifested negative responses only at the site of the placebo device. At the skin sites in those subjects challenged with the clonidine device, nine showed an equivocal (0.5) reaction, while three had a score of 1.0 at first challenge. Two weeks later, at the second challenge, three subjects had equivocal reactions, and one volunteer manifested a score of 1.0 two days following removal. However, these four subjects reacted negatively when retested with the transdermal clonidine system. One additional subject had a score of 2.0 two days following removal of the second challenge, and was thought possibly to have been sensitized to the clonidine device.

Finally, to determine whether duration of wearing the clonidine delivery system would increase the number of subjects reacting to a challenge, an additional seven day challenge was performed on the 93 Group II Draize study volunteers. In this instance, systems from the same lot of clonidine devices utilized in the induction and previous two challenges were applied and worn by subjects for one week. The elapsed time period between the second and third challenges was 30 days, during which time none of the subjects were exposed to test materials.

At the end of the seven day challenge, evaluation of skin sites immediately followed removal, and again after 24 hours. Of the 93 subjects, three had equivocal reactions at removal that were absent at re-examination 24 hours later. One subject demonstrated erythema at removal and after 24 hours, and two volunteers had both erythema and induration at removal and 24-hour recheck. The subject presumed sensitized at the previous challenge had a score of 1.0 at removal, but manifested 2.0 after one day. Thus a total of four subjects may have been sensitized to a component of the clonidine device following the seven day challenge. These four volunteers were then cross-challenged with 9% clonidine in petrolatum for 48 hours, and manifested positive reactions to this test material as well.

Results

From the cumulative results of these investigations the following conclusions seem valid at this time. First, the clonidine device, and to a lesser extent, clonidine in petrolatum are modest skin irritants to a minority of subjects, similar to some commercially available skin lubricating lotions. Second, only the clonidine device induced contact sensitization; clonidine in petrolatum at varying strengths did not. Third, prolonging the duration of the induction phase (from three to five weeks) and the duration of the challenge period (from 48 hours to seven days) increased the number of subjects showing possible allergic contact dermatitis reactions four-fold (from one to four). Finally, patients sensitized by a component of the clonidine transdermal device also manifested positive skin reactions to cross-challenge with clonidine in petrolatum, even though there were no instances of sensitization to this product by itself. Thus, at this juncture it seems most likely that clonidine in conjunction with a component of the device (a reaction product such as LUE) will turn out to be the sensitizing agent.

To determine this possibility more precisely, future lymphocyte transformation testing of blood from the four reactive subjects may confirm contact sensitization. Such testing, presumably, could clarify also whether an acetaldehyde-induced clonidine derivative is the sensitizing molecule. Projected investigations will also evaluate whether varying the placement site of the clonidine device influences the incidence of sensitization. Additionally, Draize repeat-insult, challenge-testing will be performed utilizing a device virtually without acetaldehyde to observe if elimination of this substance significantly alters sensitization incidence.

Discussion

Allergic contact dermatitis is often an inconvenience, but does not routinely fall into the category of serious medical illness. Unfortunately, there is no current method of predicting in advance which patients are predisposed to such an allergic skin reaction. For sensitized patients, the occurrence of a dermatitic reaction should be anticipated each time the skin is placed in contact with the allergen. Uncommonly, one observes flare-ups at the site of previous patch administration when allergen contact occurs elsewhere on the body. Generalized skin reactions, such as maculopapular rash, manifest in a very low percentage of cases, and usually resolve uneventfully a short time after terminating exposure to the allergen. Topical corticosteroids will accelerate the recovery process, and only rarely will a week of tapered systemic steroid therapy be necessary to promote healing. Erythema multiform and exfoliative dermatitis are extremely unusual complications of contact dermatitis.

Type IV sensitization remains restricted to localized skin reactions in the overwhelming majority of cases as a contact dermatitis. Involvement of other organ systems as a consequence of allergic hypersensitization seems uncommon, although reports on the quantitative aspects of this association are sparse. One notes only rare reports of anaphylaxis as a complication of allergic contact dermatitis; such reactions, presumably, are due to simultaneous Type I hypersensitivity.

Sixteen patients with proven topical sensitization to the clonidine device have been challenged and treated with oral clonidine for varying periods of up to one year. One of these patients developed a generalized maculopapular rash. Of note, this patient had marked renal impairment with plasma clonidine levels significantly above the normal therapeutic range (Lowenthal 1984). Moreover, 10 years of therapeutic experience with oral clonidine has not uncovered any instances of anaphylactic reactions (Maibach 1984). For these reasons, we conclude that a severe systemic reaction to oral clonidine exposure in transdermally sensitized patients will prove to be rare, or non-existent.

References

1. Boekhorst J (1983) Allergic Contact Dermatitis with Transdermal Clonidine. Lancet 2: 1031–1032
2. Groth H et al (1983) Allergic Skin Reactions to Transdermal Clonidine. Lancet 2: 850–851
3. Lowenthal D (1984) Internal communication. Boehringer-Ingelheim Ltd
4. Maibach H (1984) Clonidine Transdermal Delivery System: Cutaneous Toxicity Studies. Data on file, Boehringer-Ingelheim Ltd
5. Wilkinson DS et al (1970) Terminology of Contact Dermatitis. Acta Derm Venereol 50: 2871

Author's address:
Howard Maibach, M.D.
Department of Dermatology
University of California
School of Medicine, Moffitt Hospital
San Francisco, California 94143
U.S.A.

Transdermal Clonidine in Essential Hypertension: Problems During Long-Term Treatment

H. Groth[1], H. Vetter[3], J. Knüsel[2], P. Baumgart[3] and W. Vetter[1]

Introduction

Transdermal therapeutic systems (TTS) represent a new approach of drug administration (Shaw and Urquhart 1981, Zaffaroni 1978). These drug delivery systems are designed to release any given drug at a programmed rate, which then can be absorbed from the intact skin and thus continuously flows into the general circulation.

Compared with an equipotent oral therapy, three major advantages are possible:
1. Steady-state plasma levels over prolonged periods of time.
2. Fewer adverse-effects because of less drug-input to the body.
3. A more convenient route of drug administration which may increase patient compliance.

To date, transdermal therapeutic systems with nitroglycerine or scopolamine have proved clinically effective in the treatment of angina pectoris, motion sickness or in patients with duodenal ulcers (Georgopoulos et al. 1982; Graybiel et al. 1982; Thompson 1983; Walt et al. 1982).

Another drug suitable for transdermal application is the antihypertensive agent clonidine. Its pharmacological properties (low molecular weight, high lipid solubility, good effectiveness even at small doses) make a clonidine transdermal therapeutic system (clonidine-TTS) practical (Dollery et al. 1976; Shaw and Urquhart 1981).

Several recent studies have demonstrated a good effect using this new approach in the treatment of essential hypertension (Groth et al. 1983a; Popli et al. 1983; Weber et al. 1984). However, all these trials have had only short study periods with small numbers of patients treated at each centre. Furthermore, local skin reactions, which complicated the follow-up in up to 38% of the patients, have been reported (Groth et al. 1983b; MacMahon and Weber 1983). Whether a wider use of transdermal clonidine will be complicated by contact allergies in many patients can only be determined after analysing greater numbers of patients under treatment for months, even over years.

Patients and Methods

Clonidine-TTS, a transdermal therapeutic system containing clonidine, is a multilayer laminate 3.5 cm² in area and 200 μm thick. The system comprises a drug reservoir of either 2.5 mg (clonidine-TTS 1) or 5.0 mg (clonidine-TTS 2) clonidine surrounded by an impermeable backing membrane and a microporous membrane which guarantees a con-

Departments of Internal Medicine[1] and Dermatology[2], University Hospital, Zurich, Switzerland, and Medizinische Universitätsklinik[3], Münster, F.R.G.

stant drug release into the skin. It is fastened to the body by an adhesive layer, which also acts as a reservoir for the priming dose of clonidine. The microporous control membrane allows clonidine to be released at a constant rate of either 0.1 mg (clonidine-TTS 1) or 0.2 mg (clonidine-TTS 2)/24 h at a steady rate for at least seven days. The patches were worn on the anterior surface of the upper arm and were changed by the patients themselves once a week. The patients were instructed to affix the new transdermal delivery device to the skin of the opposite arm at each weekly change.

Thirty-five essential hypertensives (11 women, 24 men) were studied long-term, none of whom had a history of atopia. The study was approved by our local Human Study Committees and written consent was given by all subjects before entering the trial.

After a wash-out period of two weeks in all treated hypertensives, each patient received one placebo-TTS for one week. It was replaced by clonidine-TTS 1 at the end of the first week. Patients who showed a good antihypertensive response (diastolic blood pressure < 95 mmHg) remained on this treatment. Non-responders (diastolic blood pressure > 95 mmHg) received clonidine-TTS 2 from the second week on. If blood pressure control was repeatedly insufficient at subsequent controls hydrochlorothiazide (50 mg/day orally) was administered as a second drug.

Blood pressure, heart rate, and body weight were determined in weekly intervals during the dose-finding period and afterwards monthly. Blood pressure was measured with a Gelman-Hawskley-Random-Zero-Sphygmomanometer after 10 minutes of rest in a sitting position. Clonidine-typical systemic side-effects were evaluated during each visit by an analogue scale covering fatigue, nightmares, dry mouth, dizziness, Raynaud's phenomenon, obstipation, sexual disturbances and postural hypotension. Cutaneous compatibility of transdermal clonidine was supervised by a dermatologist. Patients who complained of severe systemic side-effects or intolerable local skin reactions with erythema, papules and itching etc. were withdrawn from the study. Allergy investigation procedures such as patch testing, skin biopsies or an oral rechallenge with clonidine were performed in all subjects withdrawn from the study because of skin incompatibilities.

Statistical analyses were performed by paired and unpaired Student's t-test. Differences were considered statistically significant if $p < 0.05$.

Results

Blood pressure response

Within four weeks mean blood pressure was reduced from $164 \pm 14/108 \pm 6$ to $144 \pm 12/91 \pm 6$ mmHg (P < 0.005) while treatment with placebo-TTS produced no significant blood pressure changes (Fig. 1). The therapeutic goal (diastolic blood pressure < 95 mmHg) was achieved with clonidine-TTS 1 in seven patients (20%) and 16 patients (46%) required clonidine-TTS 2. Additional therapy with 50 mg hydrochlorothiazide was necessary in the remaining 12 patients (24%). Altogether, this therapeutic regimen enabled sufficient blood pressure control in 31 of our 35 patients (89%). Patients who responded to clonidine-TTS 1, had significantly lower pretreatment blood pressure values ($155 \pm 11/102 \pm 4$ mmHg) than those with clonidine-TTS 2 plus hydrochlorothiazide ($168 \pm 12/110 \pm 6$) (p < 0.02). No major differences were observed between patients who responded to clonidine-TTS 1 or 2 ($155 \pm 11/102 \pm 4$ vs $160 \pm 7/107 \pm 5$ mmHg). Mean heart rate or mean body weight were of no discriminatory value.

Fig. 1. Systolic and diastolic blood pressure (mean ± SD) during long-term treatment with clonidine-TTS. *p < 0.005.

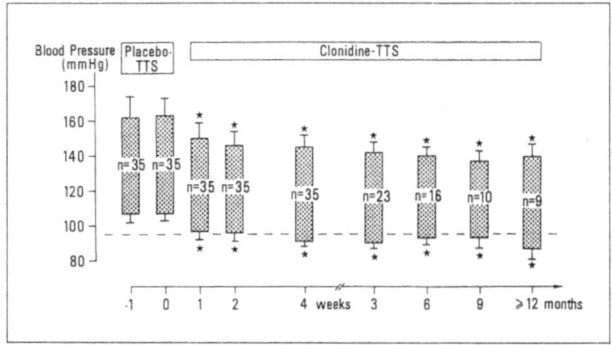

Duration of treatment

All 35 patients completed the dose-finding period. During a follow-up period of up to 22 months, no declining effectiveness of transdermal clonidine was observed in any of our patients (Fig. 1). Duration of treatment exceeded six months in 18 patients (51%). Two groups each of seven patients were treated for six to 12 or 12 to 18 months, respectively. Four patients received transdermal clonidine for 18 to 24 months.

Systemic side-effects

Twelve patients (34%) reported minor or moderate clonidine typical side-effects, such as dry mouth (n = 9), fatigue (n = 4), sexual disturbances (n = 2), Raynaud's phenomenon (n = 2), nightmares (n = 1), and obstipation (n = 1). They were observed only in patients receiving clonidine-TTS 2 with the exception of two cases. All these untoward effects occurred in the beginning of the study and resolved spontaneously during the follow-up. In one further patient, transdermal clonidine had to be discontinued after eight weeks because of a sudden onset of intolerable nightmares, fatigue and dry mouth. Determination of the plasma clonidine level on the day of withdrawal revealed three times higher values than expected. Three weeks later, treatment with clonidine-TTS 2 was again initiated and well-tolerated.

Local skin reactions

Local skin reactions were observed in 15 of our 35 patients (43%). They appeared first after at least four weeks' treatment (mean 7.8 weeks). One patient tolerated transdermal clonidine for as long as 22 weeks when suddenly a local irritation under the contact area of the patch developed. In 11 of these 15 cases the cutaneous incompatibilities increased within a few days (spreading erythema, severe itching, vesiculation and/or infiltration) and thus made a further transdermal clonidine application no longer practical. Fig. 2 shows a typical example of such a local irritation. Mild erythema with no or tolerable pruritus developed in the remaining four patients. These cases were left on clonidine-TTS. Meanwhile two of them were treated for longer than 15 months without any signs of increasing allergy.

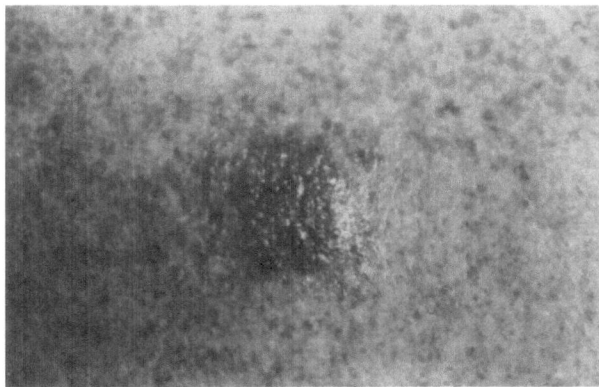

Fig. 2. Severe itching, erythema and papules after a treatment period of six weeks (♀, 46 yrs.). Subsequent patch-testing made a clonidine allergy responsible.

Allergy investigation procedures

Patch testing with all components of clonidine-TTS was performed in 10 cases who were removed from the study because of local skin problems. All patients showed a positive response to a patch containing clonidine-TTS as a whole (Table 1). In seven of these subjects allergic contact dermatitis to pure clonidine-base could be identified, whereas a contact dermatitis to another component of clonidine-TTS (polyisobutylene) turned out to be the causal agent in one patient.

Skin biopsies, which were performed in three cases, showed a fibrinous exsudate in the epidermis and lymphohistiocytic infiltration of the stratum papillare and reticulare. Four patients with positive reactions to clonidine in the patch-testing were orally rechallenged with 0.25 mg clonidine/day over 14 days. A "flare-up" phenomenon with erythema and mild itching at a former contact area with clonidine-TTS was experienced by one patient. Generalised skin reactions or systemic allergic symptoms were not observed.

Table 1. Results of patch-testing in 10 hypertensives withdrawn from clonidine-TTS treatment because of local skin reactions.

Material analysed by patch-testing	Significant response after 48–96 h
Clonidine-TTS	10 (100%)
0.5% Clonidine-base	7
Polyisobutylene	1

Discussion

In the present study it is clearly demonstrated that transdermal clonidine produced an effective and lasting reduction of blood pressure over prolonged periods of time. This new approach of drug administration enabled us in two thirds of our 35 mild or moderate essential hypertensive patients to normalise their blood pressure with clonidine-TTS 1 or 2 as monotherapy. Therefore its effectiveness is well comparable with conventional oral clonidine or other first-choice antihypertensive drugs (Frishman et al. 1979; Weber et al. 1984). However, in contrast to other recently published data with similar success rates, we found local skin reaction in 43% (n = 15) of our 35 patients (MacMahon and Weber 1983; Popli et al. 1983). An increasing pruritus, a spreading erythema, papules and an infiltration under the contact area with the patch made in most of these cases a further transdermal treatment impossible. Allergy investigation procedures such as patch-testing, skin biopsies and oral rechallenge with clonidine identified pure clonidine as the causing agent in seven of 10 studied subjects. The potential risk to induce an allergy by chronic transdermal drug administration is already well-known from other commonly used drugs (Menne and Andersen 1977; Prystowsky et al. 1979; Rasmussen and Fisher 1976; Sewing 1982). Furthermore, it is of practical importance that every subsequent oral therapy with such a drug bears the risk to develop systemic or generalised skin reactions up to the erythroderma-syndrome. Such complications are well-known from antibiotics as well as other widely used drugs (Cronin 1972; Ekenvall and Forsbeck 1978; Maibach 1975). The "flare-up" phenomenon after oral rechallenge in one of our patients indicates the possiblility of such threatening complications in subjects sensitized to clonidine. Although systemic side-effects are minor in transdermal drug therapy, an accidental uncontrolled drug release may be responsible for a sudden onset of severe systemic side-effects. This occurred in one of our patients.

In conclusion, our long-term results show a sustained and effective antihypertensive action of transdermal clonidine. However, an extremely high incidence of skin allergies, especially against clonidine, make a wider use of transdermal clonidine impractical.

References

1. Cronin E (1972) Reactions to contact allergens given orally or systemically. Brit J Derm 86: 104–107
2. Dollery CT, Davies DS, Draffan GH, Dargie HJ, Dean CR, Reid JL, Clare RA, Murray S (1976) Clinical pharmacology and pharmacokinetics of clonidine. Clin Pharmacol Ther 19: 11–17
3. Ekenvall L, Forsbeck M (1978) Contact eczema produced by a β-adrenergic blocking agent (alprenolol). Contact Dermatitis 4: 190–194
4. Frishman W, Silverman R (1979) Clinical pharmacology of the new beta-adrenergic blocking drugs. Part 3. Comparative clinical experience and new therapeutic applications. Am Heart J 98: 119–131
5. Georgopoulos AJ, Markis A, Georgiadis H (1982) Therapeutic efficacy of a new transdermal system containing nitroglycerin in patients with angina pectoris. Europ J Clin Pharmacol 22: 481–485
6. Graybiel A, Cramer DB, Wood CD (1982) Antimotion-sickness efficacy of scopolamine 12 and 72 hours after transdermal administration. Aviat Space Environ Med 53: 770–772
7. Groth H, Vetter H, Knüsel J, Boerlin HJ, Walger P, Baumgart P, Wehling M, Siegenthaler W, Vetter W (1983a) Clonidine through the skin in the treatment of essential hypertension: is it practical? J Hypertension 1 (Suppl. 2): 120–122
8. Groth H, Vetter H, Knüsel J, Vetter W (1983 b) Allergic skin reactions to transdermal clonidine. Lancet 2: 850–851
9. MacMahon FG, Weber MA (1983) Allergic skin reactions to transdermal clonidine. Lancet 2: 851
10. Maibach H (1975) Acute laryngeal obstruction presumed secondary to thiomersal (merthiolate) delayed hypersensitivity. Contact Dermatitis 1: 221–222
11. Menne T, Andersen KE (1977) Allergic contact dermatitis from fluocortolone, fluocortolone pivalate and fluocortolone caproate. Contact Dermatitis 3: 337–340

12. Popli S, Stroka G, Ing TS, Daugirdas JT, Norusis MJ, Hano JE, Gandhi VC (1983) Transdermal clonidine for hypertensive patients. Clin Ther 5: 624–628
13. Prystowsky SD, Allen AM, Smith RW, Nonomura JH, Odom RB, Akers WA (1979) Allergic contact hypersensitivity to nickel, neomycin, ethylenediamine, and benzocaine. Arch Dermatol 115: 959–962
14. Rasmussen JE, Fisher AA (1976) Allergic contact dermatitis to a salicylic acid plaster. Contact Dermatitis 2: 237–238
15. Sewing K-Fr (1982) Transdermale Medikamenten-Applikation. Dtsch med Wschr 107: 603–604
16. Shaw JE, Urquhart J (1981) Transdermal drug administration – a nuisance becomes an opportunity. Br Med J 283: 875–876
17. Thompson RH (1983) The clinical use of transdermal delivery devices with nitroglycerin. Angiology 34: 23–31
18. Walt RP, Kalman CJ, Hunt RH, Misiewicz JJ (1982) Effect of transdermally administered hyoscine methobromide on nocturnal acid secretion in patients with duodenal ulcer. Br Med J 284: 1736–1738
19. Weber MA, Drayer JIM, Brewer DD, Lipson JL (1984) Transdermal continous antihypertensive therapy. Lancet 2: 9–11
20. Zaffaroni A (1978) Therapeutic systems: The key to rational drug therapy. Drug Metab Res 8: 191–221

Authors' address:
Prof. W. Vetter
Department of Internal Medicine
University Hospital
Raemistraße 100
8091 Zürich
Switzerland

Discussion

WEBER:

The last two or three papers have focused on clinical aspects of the transdermal clonidine preparation, and some emphasis has been placed on dealing with some of the clinical side-effects of this form of therapy. I believe that there is a strong interest in the many positive aspects of this type of treatment. It is therapeutically effective, and for most patients provides convenient and well tolerated therapy. But I think it is also important for us to take a careful and responsible look at the possible adverse reactions to this form of treatment, especially any dermatological problems that can arise. The transdermal clonidine probably represents the first medication to be administered in this fashion for a truly chronic condition. Thus, we do not have any obvious precedents or prior experience to draw from, and we are very much dependent on a careful analysis of the clinical experience that has been accumulated by the investigators participating in this symposium. From the papers that have already been presented I have reached two preliminary conclusions. First, there are definitely some patients who will experience skin reaction to the use of the transdermal medication. There are some differences in opinion concerning the frequency of this problem, and I suspect that we have not yet fully defined the differing forms and severities of these reactions. My second conclusion, however, is that we have not yet heard of a single case of a truly major or life-threatening complication. Nevertheless, since our experience with this new form of treatment is still relatively limited, we should at least consider some of the theoretical possibilities for serious events to occur. I should like to start this discussion by asking Dr Calnan, who has had great experience in the field of dermatological reactions to treatment, about the time-course of reactions to this type of therapy. In your paper, you suggested that immunologically mediated reactions to therapy normally take place within the first three months of treatment. Does this suggest that other factors might participate in reactions that are seen late in treatment, or is it still possible that some patients have a slower onset of the immune-type reaction?

CALNAN:

As you indicate, the time-course of these events is not always totally predictable. It can sometimes be difficult, even for experienced dermatologists, to determine the mechanism by which a skin reaction to treatment may occur.

DRAYER:

If a patient has had previous allergic reactions to another medication or to other types of antigens, would this predict the likelihood of a reaction when treatment with transdermal clonidine is administered?

CALNAN:

At this stage, I think the correct answer to your question is in the negative. I know that some investigators and some manufacturers of drugs and related products have anticipated that patients with eczema, asthma, or hay fever might be susceptible to allergic reactions, but there is no evidence that this is truly the case. There are no obvious clinical clues that are of predictive value in this context.

BOEKHORST:

If a patient has a type IV immunological reaction to the transdermal treatment, what is the likelihood of a subsequent type I reaction during treatment with oral clonidine?

CALNAN:

I believe that this chance is extremely small. As you know, type IV reactions to a fairly wide variety of drugs are very common, and dermatologists and other physicians see very large numbers of these reactions. Yet it is rare for us to see type I sensitivity reactions, even though we know that many patients continue to receive exposure to the agent that produced the original reaction. The experience with penicillin is a reasonable anology, and helps point out the difficulty in predicting reactions.

WEBER:

I should like to ask the investigators who have just published their experience with the transdermal clonidine, whether they have seen any type of generalized reaction to the treatment that would have caused serious medical concern on behalf of the patient. Have you seen anything that could be regarded as life-threatening or of major significance?

GROTH:

We have not seen any reactions of that type. We have seen only local skin reactions to the transdermal clonidine, although one patient did experience some itching and erythema upon oral rechallenge.

KELLAWAY:

Approximately 20% of our patients with the transdermal clonidine were withdrawn from the study at the end of six months. A few other patients had some minor skin reactions, but these were not of any significance and did not cause real inconvenience. We did rechallenge 10 patients who were withdrawn from the study with oral clonidine therapy. None of them had any systemic reactions.

SAMBHI:

Some studies have suggested that older individuals might be more susceptible to allergic reactions to medication than younger individuals. Could Dr Groth tell us more about the age and sex distribution of his patients who experienced skin reactions?

GROTH:

That is a good question. We looked carefully at possible characteristics of patients who had skin reactions, but we found that neither the age nor the sex of the patient could be used to predict the likelihood of their having a reaction. Moreover, there did not seem to be any association with time of year; reactions appeared to happen equally during the four seasons.

LOWENTHAL:

It has been suggested that age and an exposure to many medications and other environmental toxins may make patients more predisposed to allergic reactions. Thus, it could be anticipated, at least on theoretical grounds, that older individuals might be more vulnerable and consequently, that younger patients would have fewer reactions. In our study with the transdermal clonidine, we have been treating approximately 20 adolescent patients, with ages ranging from 11 to 18 years, for up to six months. We have seen no skin problems, and in general the patients have tolerated the treatment very well. I think that the question raised by Dr Sambhi is important, and it might be valuable to take a careful look at the combined clinical experiences with transdermal clonidine to see whether age is a factor in predicting a reaction.

WEBER:

There are obviously differences among investigators concerning the frequency of skin reactions in their patients. For example, the studies performed in the United States appeared to find a lower frequency of skin reaction than studies in Northern Europe. How important are different environments, or perhaps different types of populations, in determining the frequency of these types of reactions?

CALNAN:

It is now widely accepted that there are wide differences from one country to another in the incidence of both allergic and non-allergic adverse reactions to medications. Obvious possibilities are that racial and genetic differences might be factors in explaining the variations between countries, but there is little evidence to support this. It is more likely that the explanation lies in local environmental factors. Patients in Europe and in the United States are probably exposed to different allergens, and could thus develop different degrees of vulnerability to reactions to new medication or treatment.

BRAVO:

It is sometimes possible that a medication can be formulated in slightly different ways depending on where it is prepared or manufactured. Is it possible that the transdermal clonidine patches being used by the investigators who have presented their papers at this meeting were made in different places or as part of separate batches?

KAPLAN:

I have carefully examined all available data, and come to the conclusion that there is no evidence that the likelihood of skin reactions has been greater following treatment with materials taken from one batch or another. Moreover, all of the skin patches have been manufactured by an identical process, and all in the one plant. We have even re-examined the origins of the raw materials used in making the skin patches, and again there appeared to be no differences.

KUCHEL:

I am not completely satisfied that we have dealt with some of the difficult questions here. There is obviously a remarkable difference in the incidence of skin reactions between some of the major centres. For example, the study presented by the Swiss investigators found a rather high incidence of this problem, whereas studies carried out in France have found virtually no adverse skin effects. Apart from some of the demographic and environmental factors that we have already discussed, could the duration of treatment given to the patients in the various studies also help explain this apparent discrepancy?

KAPLAN:

We have carefully looked at all the data from studies with the transdermal clonidine carried out in the United States, Europe and New Zealand. We found that 70% of all drop-outs from treatment caused by skin reactions occurred within 12 weeks of the start of therapy, and 90% of withdrawals from treatment had occurred by 20 weeks. Our analysis would predict that patients who do not yet have an adverse skin effect by three months have at least a 95% likelihood of reaching 12 months of treatment without such a reaction. Although two of the papers presented in this symposium did find a rather high incidence of the skin reactions, other studies have found a far lower incidence. I think some of the suggestions made by Professor Calnan and other speakers are helpful in explaining differences between the various study centres, and obviously we shall be carefully scrutinizing further data as more studies are undertaken and completed.

KOLLOCH:

We must consider questions of geography or duration of treatment as factors in the appearance of skin reactions to the transdermal clonidine treatment, but I think we should also evaluate the side-effect in terms of its seriousness. In our experience, the skin reactions are immediately noticed by the patients, chiefly through pruritis, and they tend to report this immediately to the physician. This enables the physician to make an immediate decision concerning the treatment: should he stop it, or is the complaint sufficiently mild and tolerable to allow the therapy to continue? In some ways this situation is far preferable to other side-effects with antihypertensive treatment, such as adverse metabolic changes, which might not be recognized by either the patient or the physician. I think it is important to raise the question discussed by Dr Weber earlier. Have the investigators who have studied the transdermal clonidine seen any dermatological reaction that they would classify as being truly serious or life-threatening, or are we talking about something that is an inconvenience, even if at times a somewhat unpleasant one. In the final analysis, it is important to know whether anyone can report a patient in whom lasting harm has been done.

GROTH:

Even though we have seen several patients with allergic skin reactions to the transdermal treatment, we have not seen complications that could be regarded as dangerous or life-threatening. Nevertheless, if you see a relatively high incidence of skin reactions, and have the experience of having progessively more patients complain as time goes by, it is reasonable to question whether this approach to treatment is really of value in a conventional hypertension programme. As you know, the treatment of hypertension must continue on a long-term basis in each patient, and I normally like the reassurance of knowing that a particular form of treatment will not only be effective but that it will also be well tolerated for more than just a few weeks or months.

WEBER:

Your point is well taken. If 30 or 40% of your patients have symptomatic complaints which force them to discontinue the treatment, you are entitled to be cautious in your use of this therapeutic approach on a routine basis. But the point raised by Dr Kuchel is relevant here, for many investigators did not find this high incidence of skin reactions, even in studies of relatively long duration. I think it is important that practicing clinicians be properly educated about the use and properties of the transdermal medication. They should be informed that at least some of their patients will not comfortably tolerate the treatment, and that they should be ready to switch to alternative approaches should this be necessary. After all, this is how we already deal with the various conventional forms of medication that we use for the treatment of our hypertensive patients.

DRAYER:

In an earlier symposium on the use of differing forms of transdermal medication, Kligman in the United States made the point that any area of skin that is occluded for several days by an adhesive patch is susceptible to irritation and possible sensitization. In our experience we have found it helpful in some patients to move the patch after three or four days in one position rather than waiting to replace it after the full seven days. We believe that this definitely reduces the likelihood of a skin reaction developing under the patch.

CALNAN:

Speaking as a dermatologist, I agree with the possibility that long-term occlusion of the skin increases the chance of a reaction. If it is possible to move the transdermal clonidine patch from one position to another without causing any loss of efficacy then this indeed might be a good strategy in certain patients. Clearly the best person to make this type of decision is the patient himself. Most people with high blood pressure recognize the importance of long-term treatment, and will usually have tried one or more antihypertensive drug in an attempt to control their high blood pressure. I have the strong impression that the majority of such individuals will be able to decide for themselves whether the mild skin reactions that they might experience during the transdermal treatment are more or less tolerable than side-effects they might have experienced during previous oral treatment. Since we have no evidence to suggest that there is any significant medical problem with the occurrence of skin reactions, it would seem sensible to allow the patient to determine whether the treatment with the transdermal medication should be continued or replaced.

Low Dose Oral and Transdermal Application of Clonidine in Mild Hypertension: Hemodynamic and Biochemical Correlates

R. Kolloch, H. Finster, A. Overlack, H. M. Müller, K. O. Stumpe

Introduction

The antihypertensive effect of clonidine has been demonstrated in all grades of hypertension in numerous studies (4, 6, 12, 22, 25, 26). Data on the dose-response relationship for clonidine are only available for the range from 0.300 to 0.750 mg/day (8, 10, 17). In this range, also described as a therapeutic window, there is a close relationship between the hypotensive effect and an increase of the side effects such as sedation and reduced salivation (8, 12, 17).

Pilot studies on a small number of patients indicated that even in a daily dose of less than 0.300 mg clonidine has a definite antihypertensive effect with fewer side effects and therefore a low dosage may be suitable for treating mild forms of hypertension.

Our aim was therefore to establish to what extent an antihypertensive effect with a lower incidence of side effects can be achieved with a low dosage of clonidine. The antihypertensive effect of low dose oral clonidine was compared with that of the beta-blocker metoprolol in a multi-centre study, and the effect of clonidine, administered transdermally, on hemodynamics and sympathetic activity was analysed in a second study.

Patients and Methods

Group I

Group I comprised 71 patients accepted for a multicentre double-blind study. After a 2-week control period there was a 6-week treatment period in which, allocated at random, one group of patients (n = 35) was treated with clonidine and a second group (n = 36) was treated with metoprolol. There was no difference between the two groups of patients with regard to sex, age, height, weight and pretreatment blood pressures (Table 1). In the first 3 weeks the patients were either given 0.0375 mg of clonidine b.d. or 50 mg of metoprolol b.d. If the reduction of blood pressure was inadequate after 3 weeks the dose

Medizinische Universitäts-Poliklinik Bonn, F.R.G.

Table 1. Patients of group I.

	Clonidine	Metoprolol
Number	N = 35	N = 36
Sex	21 M, 14 F	24 M, 12 F
Age (years)	53 ± 15	55 ± 15
Height (cm)	170 ± 9	170 ± 8
Weight (kg)	76 ± 12	76 ± 13

was increased to 0.075 mg of clonidine b.d. or 100 mg of metoprolol b.d. Blood pressure and pulse rate were measured after 5 minutes' supine and 2 minutes' standing, once a week.

Group II

A second group of patients was given low doses of clonidine by the transdermal therapeutic system (TTS). This system consists of a membrane covering a drug reservoir. The release of the drug to the skin is controlled by a micropore membrane to achieve constant release and absorption. Thirteen patients with mild hypertension were treated by this new technique in a placebo-controlled single-blind study. The patients' diastolic blood pressure, measured on 3 days before treatment, was between 90 and 104 mmHg. Their mean age was 46 (24 to 69) years. The patients' sodium intake was unrestricted and they showed a mean sodium excretion of 156 mEq/24 h. All the patients were treated for the first 2 weeks with the placebo-TTS and then for 4 weeks with clonidine-TTS. At first one patch was applied once a week for 2 weeks. If the reduction of blood pressure was inadequate, the patients received 2 patches per week. There were weekly controls of blood pressure, pulse rate, plasma levels of clonidine and side effects. At the end of the 2-week placebo period and after 2 and 4 weeks' treatment with clonidine-TTS we measured the noradrenaline concentration and renin activity in the plasma and the excretion of noradrenaline, kallikrein, sodium and potassium in the 24 h urine. The glomerular filtration rate was calculated from the endogenous creatinine clearance.

The effect of clonidine-TTS on the blood pressure during isometric handgrip exercise was also analysed. The patients compressed a hand dynamometer for 3 minutes using one-third of their maximum voluntary contraction. Before the start and at the end of the exercise we measured the blood pressure and pulse rate and again determined the noradrenaline concentration and renin activity in the plasma.

The urinary sodium concentration was determined with a laboratory flame photometer and the plasma and urinary creatinine concentration was determined with an auto-analyser.

Noradrenaline was measured by a sensitive radio-enzymatic technique (7) and the plasma renin activity and clonidine concentration were measured by radio-immunoassay (2, 14).

In group I the statistical analysis involved an analysis of variance for a three-factor model and multiple comparisons by the Scheffé test. In group II the results were analysed by the paired Student t-test. Unless stated otherwise, the data are expressed as mean values ± standard deviation.

Results

Group I

After one week a daily dose of 0.075 mg of clonidine orally resulted in a significant reduction ($p < 0.05$) of the systolic and diastolic blood pressure. As the treatment continued the hypotensive effect increased. After 6 weeks' treatment the blood pressure had fallen from $160 \pm 13/93 \pm 9$ mmHg to $141 \pm 12/84 \pm 6$ mmHg ($p < 0.001$) (Fig. 1). In the patients given 50 mg of metoprolol b.d. after 6 weeks' treatment the blood pressure had fallen from $159 \pm 10/95 \pm 8$ mmHg to $140 \pm 13/84 \pm 5$ mmHg ($p < 0.001$) (Fig. 1).

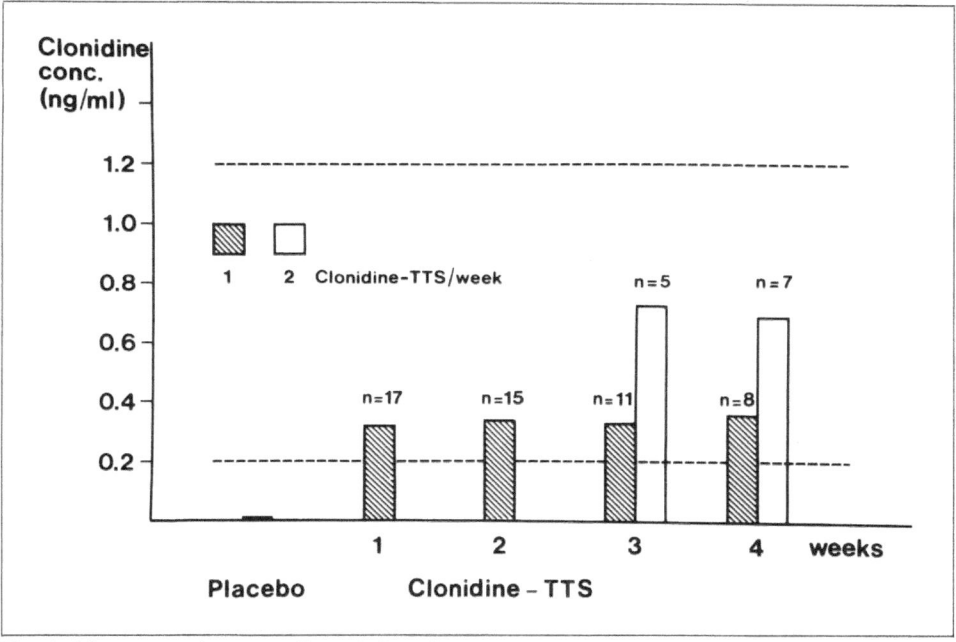

Fig. 1. Mean recumbent systolic and diastolic pressure and heart rate readings before and during treatment with 0.0375 mg of clonidine b.d. or 50 mg of metoprolol b.d.

There was only a minimal reduction of the pulse rate under the low dose of clonidine, whereas the reduction of the pulse rate was rather more pronounced under metoprolol (Fig. 1).

With the low dosage there were very few side effects in the two groups. Four of 35 patients treated with clonidine reported such side effects as slight tiredness (n = 3) and mild sleep disturbances (n = 1). None of the patients complained of a dry mouth. There were side effects in 2 of the 36 patients treated with metoprolol, these being slight tiredness and a slight feeling of lethargy. In both groups the side effects diminished as the treatment progressed.

Group II

The mean plasma levels of clonidine with an application of one clonidine patch per week were 0.3 ng/ml. The mean plasma levels of clonidine doubled on average when the dose was increased to 2 patches per week. Overall, the clonidine plasma levels indicate that absorption of the drug was continuous and uniform throughout the observation period (Fig. 2). As regards the hypotensive effect of clonidine-TTS, 2 of the 13 patients treated were non-responders; these were defined as patients in whom the fall of diastolic pressure was $\leqslant 5$ mmHg. The blood pressure was controlled satisfactorily in 7 of the 11 responders with one patch a week and in 4 patients with 2 patches a week.

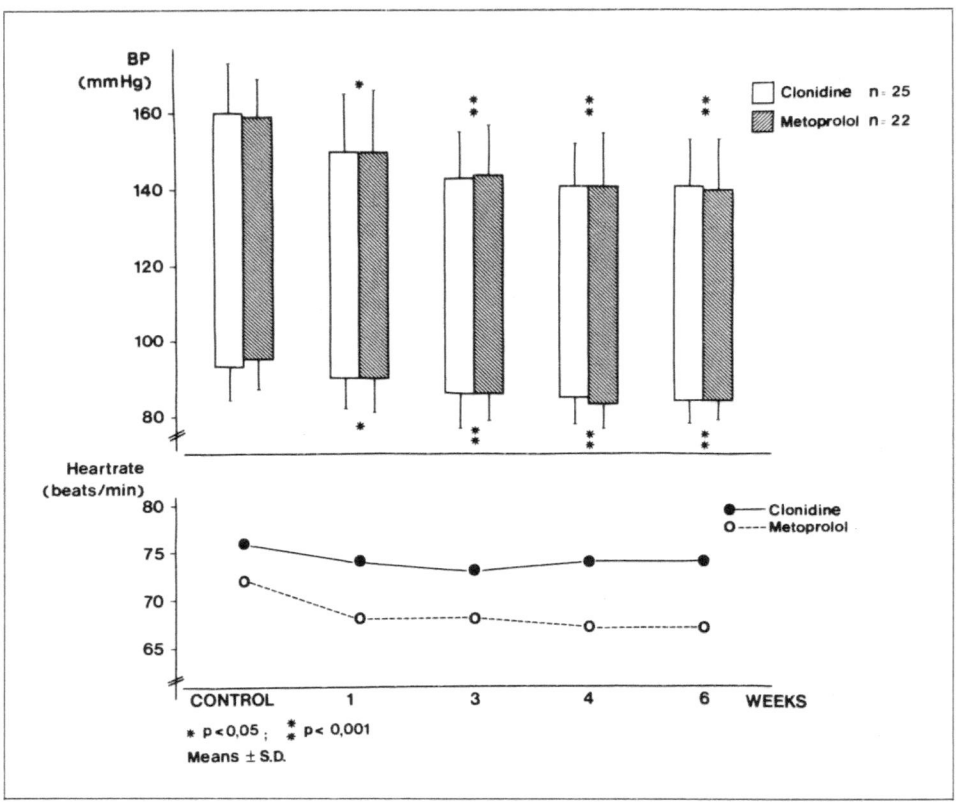

Fig. 2. Plasma concentration of clonidine with application of 1 and 2 clonidine patches per week. The broken lines show the range of the "therapeutic window" for clonidine.

Figure 3 shows the blood pressure and pulse rate during treatment in the 11 responders. There was a significant reduction of the systolic and diastolic blood pressure in the supine and standing position. There was only a minor effect on the pulse rate.

After 4 weeks' treatment the plasma noradrenaline concentration decreased from 488 to 335 ng/l and the urinary excretion of noradrenaline fell from 20.6 to 13.1 μg/24 h ($p < 0.001$) (Fig. 4).

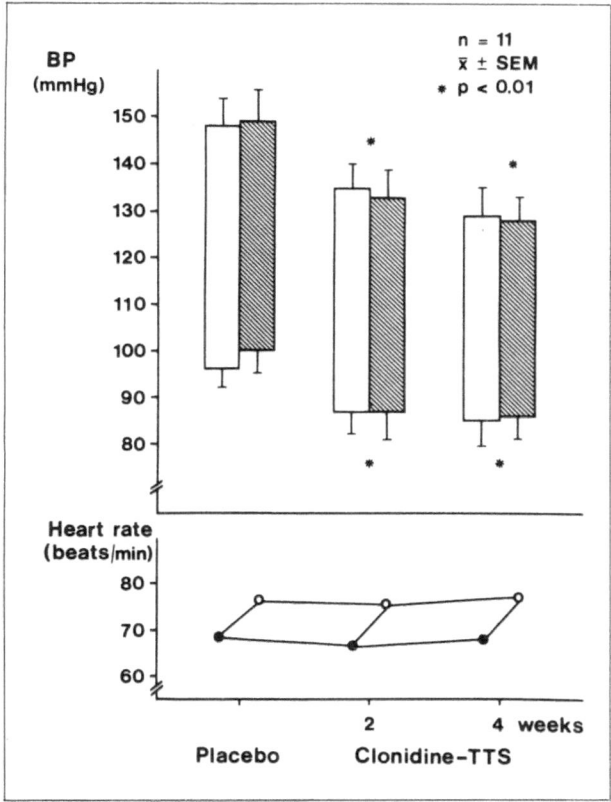

Fig. 3. Effect of clonidine-TTS on the systolic and diastolic pressure supine (open bars) and standing (hatched bars) and the pulse rate supine (solid circles) and standing (open circles) in the 11 responders.

During isometric handgrip exercise the plasma noradrenaline concentration under the placebo rose from 488 to 587 ng/l. After 2 weeks' clonidine-TTS treatment the plasma noradrenaline concentration rose from 391 to 488 ng/l and after 4 weeks from 335 to 434 ng/l. Whereas the resting values were depressed during clonidine-TTS treatment the absolute responsiveness as regards stimulation of the release of noradrenaline remained largely unchanged. The percentage change of the plasma noradrenaline concentration during isometric handgrip exercise increased minimally but not significantly during clonidine-TTS treatment (Fig. 5).

During the placebo-TTS, handgrip raised the systolic (17%) and diastolic (20%) pressure, the pulse rate (12%) as well as the plasma noradrenaline concentration (20%) and plasma renin activity (22%). After the blood pressure had been restored to normal and the sympathetic tone suppressed by clonidine-TTS, the percentage responsiveness remained unchanged during physical exercise (Fig. 6).

After 2 weeks' treatment with clonidine-TTS mean sodium excretion had risen from 156 to 176 mEq/24 h (p < 0.05). The glomerular filtration rate and kallikrein excretion with the 24 h urine did not change during treatment.

Clonidine-TTS was very well tolerated. Subjective and local side effects throughout the observation period were minimal and only transient. There were no discernible changes in the clinical chemistry parameters. Clonidine-TTS had no effect on the lipid profile after either 2 or 4 weeks' use.

Fig. 4. Significant reduction of the plasma noradrenaline concentration and of noradrenaline excretion in the 24 h urine during 2 weeks and 4 weeks of clonidine-TTS treatment.

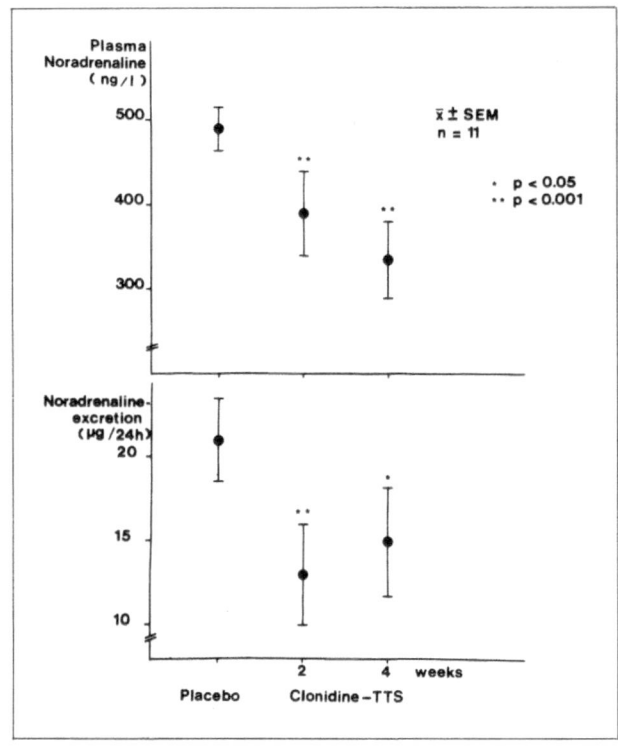

Fig. 5. Absolute and percentage change in the plasma noradrenaline concentration during isometric handgrip exercise. After clonidine-TTS the stimulation of the sympathetic activity during physical exercise was maintained.

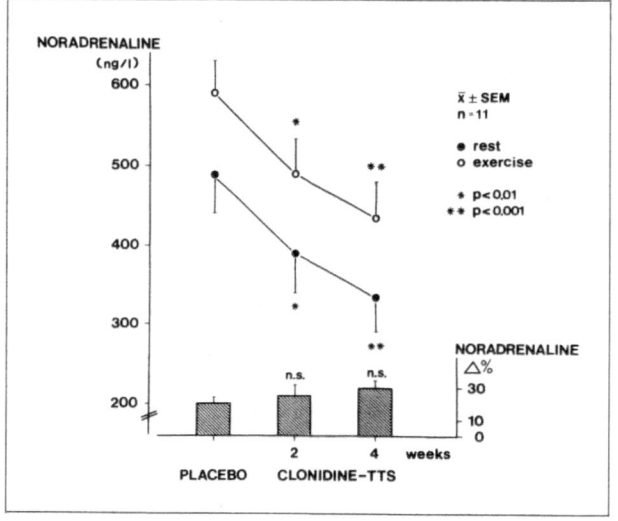

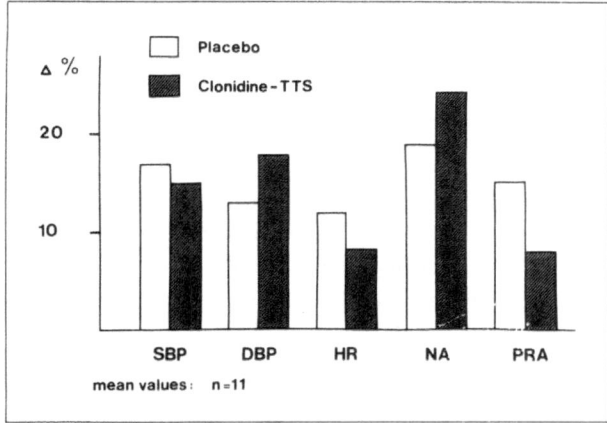

Fig. 6. Effect of clonidine-TTS on systolic pressure (SBP), diastolic pressure (DBP), heart rate (HR), noradrenaline (NA) and plasma renin activity (PRA) during isometric exercise. None of the parameters show any significant change in their percentage responsiveness to stimulation.

Discussion

The results of this study show that clonidine in a low oral dosage reduced the systolic and diastolic blood pressure. The hypotensive effect was comparable to that of the cardioselective beta-blocker metoprolol. There was only a minimal reduction of pulse rate under clonidine, whilst the reduction of pulse rate was more pronounced under metoprolol.

With the daily dose of 0.075 to 0.150 mg there were no reports of the side effects typical of clonidine, such as dry mouth or pronounced tiredness.

With low-dosed trandermal application of clonidine too there was a definite antihypertensive effect with a low incidence of side effects.

Recent studies on normotensive volunteers have shown that after single oral doses of 0.075, 0.150 and 0.250 mg of clonidine there is a dose-related increase of the hypotensive effect and of the frequency and severity of sedation and dry mouth (1, 8). As a rule, side effects occur 1 to 2 hours after dosing and, with higher dosages, they persist for up to 8 hours (1). With the dose of 0.0375 mg b.d. which we selected there were no appreciable side effects. Even when the dose was increased to 0.075 mg of clonidine b.d. in patients in whom the reduction of blood pressure had been inadequate there was no increase of the side effects, indicating that tolerance develops with long-term treatment.

With 1 clonidine-TTS patch a week the mean clonidine concentration was 0.3 ng/ml. This was roughly the same as the plasma concentrations found with daily oral administration of 0.050 mg b.d. or 0.0375 mg of clonidine b.d. (Frisk-Holmberg, personal communication).

The average plasma concentration of clonidine doubled when the clonidine-TTS dose was increased to 2 patches a week. Overall, there was continuous and constant transdermal absorption of clonidine with largely constant mean plasma concentrations. The clonidine concentrations found with transdermal administration were therefore in the lower range of the "therapeutic window" of 0.2 to 1.2 ng/ml. With dosages which produce plasma concentrations above 1.2 ng of clonidine/ml, it is thought possible that the antihypertensive effect is reduced due to stimulation of peripheral alpha-adrenergic receptors (10, 12).

The favourable relationship between hypotensive effect and incidence of side effects found in our studies with low oral or transdermal doses indicates that, contrary to earlier recommendations, used in a correspondingly low dose, clonidine could also be suitable for patients with mild hypertension.

The hypotensive effect of clonidine is ascribed primarily to its inhibitory action on central and peripheral sympathetic nervous system activity (15, 18, 27). Numerous studies have demonstrated suppression of the plasma noradrenaline concentration with fairly high doses of clonidine (16, 28). There are as yet no data available on sympathetic activity during long-term low-dosed clonidine treatment of patients with essential hypertension. The dose-related suppression of the plasma noradrenaline concentration and the reduction of noradrenaline excretion in the 24 h urine found in our study indicate that even with very low doses of clonidine the hypotensive effect is mediated by a reduction of sympathetic tone, and that even minimal doses of clonidine are sufficient to inhibit the sympathetic nervous system.

Clonidine-TTS had little effect on the heart rate, indicating that the reduction of heart rate observed under higher doses of clonidine may contribute little to its hypotensive effect.

The effect of antihypertensive treatment on the blood pressure during exercise is also a factor to be considered when deciding whether blood pressure control is satifactory. We therefore analysed the effect of isometric handgrip exercise on hemodynamics and on biochemical parameters during clonidine-TTS administration.

Isometric or static exercise is frequently performed during a normal day's activity, including lifting, carrying, holding pushing, pulling or raising the intraabdominal pressure. Compression of a hand dynamometer with 30% of maximum voluntary contraction is roughly equivalent to carrying 10 kg in one hand. This level of work is performed by many patients briefly several times a day. In hypertensive patients isometric exercise immediately raises the heart rate and systolic and diastolic pressure and represents a potential hazard to this group of patients (19, 21). The rise of blood pressure is associated with a significant rise of plasma catecholamines and the sympathetic nervous system appears to play an important role in mediating the cardiovascular changes observed (19, 20, 21). The effect of antihypertensive drugs on the response to exercise during isometric strain has not been adequately investigated. For example, an excessive rise of blood pressure during isometric exercise has been demonstrated in hypertensive patients being treated with the beta-blocker propranolol (21). Our results during treatment with the placebo-TTS indicate that noradrenaline release and the cardiovascular system are stimulated during isometric muscular work. During clonidine-TTS treatment there was suppression or normalization of the sympathetic tone and of the elevated blood pressure under resting conditions, whilst the normal response to exercise, i.e. the physiological responsiveness to stimulation, remained intact.

The interrelationship of sympathetic nervous activity and the sodium-volume balance on the one hand and renal function on the other have been investigated recently (5, 9, 11). There are conflicting results regarding the effect of clonidine on renal function and the sodium balance (5, 24). After 2 weeks' treatment with clonidine-TTS we observed an increase of sodium excretion, which subsequently returned to the pretreatment values. Since we did not monitor the metabolic balance continuously in our patients, we cannot conclude from these data that the sodium balance was negative at the beginning of treatment. These results, together with the fact that the body weight remained constant, at least refute the possibility of appreciable sodium and water retention during clonidine-TTS administration.

The possibility that anithypertensive drugs alter the lipid profile and thus increase the risk of cardiovascular disease has attracted increasing interest in recent years. Our results show that clonidine-TTS did not cause any changes whatsoever in the lipid profile during the 4-week observation period.

Our patients showed no appreciable local side effects during the 4-week period of treatment with clonidine-TTS. However, localized skin reactions with pruritus, erythema, vesiculation and/or inflammatory infiltrates have been reported with varying frequency by us and other authors with fairly long-term use (13, 23). More data from larger groups of patients are mandatory to assess the long-term skin tolerance to clonidine-TTS and the clinical relevance of the allergic skin reactions observed.

In summary our results show that, given orally in a dose of 0.0375 to 0.075 mg b.d., clonidine has a definite hypotensive effect comparable to that of the beta-blocker metoprolol in a dosage of 50 to 100 mg b.d. There were no appreciable side effects in this dose range. Even with low-dosed transdermal administration clonidine exhibited a definite hypotensive effect and at the same time it reduced sympathetic tone. When clonidine-TTS had restored the blood pressure to normal and suppressed the sympathetic nervous system the responsiveness to stimulation during physical exercise remained intact. The plasma levels of clonidine indicate that the drug was absorbed continuously and uniformly through the skin. Subjective and local side effects during the treatment period were minor and only transient. There were no untoward changes in serum lipids. The good acceptance by the patients indicates that the weekly transdermal administration of clonidine may improve patient compliance in the treatment of mild essential hypertension.

Acknowledgements

We would like to thank Miss M. Higuchi, Dr. J. Yadel, Miss M. Lennarz and Miss Ch. Ressel for their expert assistance in performing the biochemical analyses, and Mrs. L. Mehrem for her secretarial help.

References

1. Anavekar SN, Jarrott B, Toscano M, Louis J (1982) Pharmacokinetic and pharmacodynamic studies of oral clonidine in normotensive subjects. Europ J Clin Pharm 23: 1–5
2. Arndt SD, Stähle H, Förster HJ (1981) Development of a RIA for clonidine and its comparison with the reference methods. J Pharmacol Methods 6: 298
3. Barr JG, Kauker ML (1979) Renal tubular site and mechanism of clonidine-induced diuresis in rats: clearance and micropuncture studies. J Pharmacol Exp Ther 209: 389
4. Bock KD, Merguet P, Heimsoth VH (1973) Effect of clonidine on regional blood flow and its use in the treatment of hypertension. In: Onesti G, Kim KE, Moyer JH (eds) 26th Hahneman Symposium: Hypertension Mechanisms and Management Grune & Stratton, New York pp 395–403
5. Campese VM (1983) Natrium und Volumenbilanz bei Hypertonikern und Clonidin. In: Hayduk K, Bock KD (Hrsg) Zentrale Blutdruckregulation durch alpha 2-Rezeptorenstimulation. Steinkopff Verlag Darmstadt S 90
6. Chalemphol T, Golub MS, Eggena P, Barrett JD, Sambhi MP (1982) Clonidine, a centrally acting sympathetic inhibitor, as monotherapy for mild to moderate hypertension. Am J Cardiol 49: 153
7. DaPrada M, Zurcher G (1976) Simultaneous radioenzymatic determination of plasma and tissue adrenaline, noradrenaline and dopamine within the femtomole range. Life Sci 19: 1161
8. Davies DS, Wing LMH, Reid JL, Neill E, Tippett P, Dollery CT (1977) Pharmacokinetics and concentration-effect relationships of intravenous and oral clonidine. Clin Pharmacol Ther 21: 593–601

9. Dibona GF (1977) Neurogenic regulation of renal tubular sodium reabsorption. Am J Physiol 233: F 73
10. Dollery CT, Davies DS, Draffan GH, Dargie HJ, Dean CR, Reid JL, Clare RA, Murray S (1976) Clinical pharmacology and pharmacokinetics of clonidine. Clin Pharmacol Ther 19: 11–17
11. Fink GD, Brody MJ (1978) Continuous measurement of renal blood flow changes to renal nerve stimulation and intra-arterial drug administration in the rat. Am J Physiol 234: H 219
12. Frisk-Holmberg M (1980) The Effectiveness of Clonidine as an Antihypertensive in a Two-Dose Regimen. Acta Med Scand 207: 43–45
13. Groth H, Vetter H, Knüsel J, Vetter W (1983) Allergic skin reactions to transdermal clonidine. Lancet II 850
14. Haber E et al (1969) Application of radioimmunoassay for angiotensin I to the physiologic measurements of plasma renin activity in normal human subjects. J Clin Endocrinol Metab 29: 1349
15. Haeusler G (1974) Clonidine-induced inhibition of sympathetic nerve activity: No indication for a central presynaptic of an indirect sympathomimetic mode of action. Naunyn-Schmiedebergs Arch Pharmacol 286: 97
16. Hofkelt B, Hedeland H, Dymling JF (1970) Studies on catecholamines, renin and aldosterone following Catapresan (2-(2,6-Dichlor-Phenylamine)-2-imidazoline Hydrochloride) in hypertensive patients. Eur J Pharmacol 10: 389
17. Keränen AS, Nykänen J, Tashinen J (1978) Pharmacokinetics and side-effects of clonidine. Europ J Clin Pharmacol 13: 97
18. Kobinger W, Walland W (1972) Facilitation of vagal reflex bradykardia by an action of clonidine on central alpha receptors. Europ J Pharmacol 9: 210
19. Kolloch R, Meyers M, Bornheimer J, DcQuattro V (1981) Hämodynamik und Plasmakatecholamine während statistischer Muskelarbeit bei essentieller Hypertonie. Verh Dtsch Ges Inn Med 87: 533
20. Martin CE et al (1974) Autonomic mechanisms in hemodynamic responses to isometric exercise. J Clin Invest 54: 104
21. McAllister RG (1979) Effect of adrenergic receptor blockade on the responses to isometric handgrip: studies in normal and hypertensive subjects. J Cardiovasc Pharmacol 1: 253–263
22. McMahon FG (1978) Management of Essential Hypertension. Futura, New York
23. McMahon FG, Weber AM (1983) Allergic skin reactions to transdermal clonidine. Lancet II, 851
24. Olsen UB (1976) Clonidine induced increase of renal prostaglandin activity and water diuresis in conscious dogs. Eur J Pharmacol 36: 95
25. Onesti G, Schwartz AB, Kim KE, Paz-Martinez V, Swartz C (1971) Antihypertensive effect of clonidine. Circ Res 28, 29 (Suppl 2): 53
26. Pettinger WA (1975) Clonidine, a new antihypertensive drug. New Engl J Med 293: 1179
27. Schmit H (1977) The pharmacology of clonidine and related products. In: Antihypertensive Agents. Gross F (ed), Springer-Verlag Berlin, Heidelberg, New York pp 299–396
28. Wing LHM, Reid JL, Hamilton A, Sever P, Davies DS, Dollery CT (1977) Effects of clonidine on biochemical indices of sympathetic and plasma renin activity in normotensive man. Clin Sci 53: 45

Authors' address:
Dr. R. Kolloch
Medizinische Universitäts-Poliklinik
Wilhelmstraße 35–37
5300 Bonn 1
F.R.G.

Regression of Left Ventricular Hypertrophy in Nineteen Hypertensive Patients Treated with Clonidine for Eighteen Months: A Prospective Study

F. Gilbert McMahon, Ronald Michael, Jerome R. Ryan, William St. John LaCorte, and Adesh Jain

Introduction

Echocardiography provides a relatively simple, non-invasive, reproducible means of assessing left ventricular hypertrophy (LVH). Evidence has accumulated both from animal and clinical studies that LVH occurs quite early as a cardiac response to hypertension and indeed occurs at a greater frequency (40–50% of mild to moderate cases) than had been previously anticipated by electrocardiographic studies (2–5%) of similarly hypertensive patients. Recent studies also indicate that LVH can regress, with appropriate drug therapy, within a relatively short interval of time, but whether or not this is accompanied by reversal of vascular hypertrophy or by salubrious or adverse effects of ventricular function and coronary blood flow is not established. A variety of antihypertensive medications have been studied in an effort to reverse LVH. It appears that drugs which inhibit catecholamines, e.g., α_2-agonists, converting enzyme inhibitors and β-blocking agents, are capable of reducing LVH at least in many patients. On the other hand, drugs which increase catecholamines, such as diuretics and direct vasodilators, appear to have no beneficial effect on LVH in spite of satisfactory reductions in blood pressure.

We decided to investigate the long-term effects of a fixed combination of clonidine given together with chlorthalidone as Combipres in a group of patients with established essential hypertension and clear LVH by both electrographic voltage criteria, as well as echocardiographic measurements.

Patients and Methods

Twenty hypertensive patients were enrolled, but one was removed from the study early on for personal reasons. There were six males and 13 females. Their mean age was 58 years (the range was 45–70 years), and their mean body weight was 180 lb (range 167–209 lb). The average duration of hypertension was 14 years (the range was 11–17 years). All had both echocardiographic (ECHO) and electrocardiographic (ECG) evidence of LVH. Patients were excluded who had child-bearing potential, clinically significant renal or hepatic disease, or who were receiving antihypertensive or other medications which affected blood pressure.

Department of Medicine of Tulane University School of Medicine and The Clinical Research Center, New Orleans, Louisiana, U.S.A.

Patients whose seated blood pressures were not adequately controlled on diuretics alone (i.e., diastolic blood pressure less than 95 mmHg) and who required additional antihypertensive therapy were given Combipres over six weeks with the dose titrated as necessary to a maximum of two tablets twice daily of Combipres (each tablet contained 0.2 mg clonidine/15 mg chlorthalidone). The study was continued for 18 months (Table 1). All patients gave written informed consent, and institutional peer review was obtained before the start of the trial. M-mode echocardiograms, recorded by the same technician and after having been coded, were read blind by an independent cardiologist uninvolved in the study. A Honeywell Ultra Imager was used with a 3.5 mgHz transducer to perform the echogram. Measurements were obtained following the recommendations of the American Society of Echocardiography. Left ventricular mass was calculated using the formula $LVM(g) = [(ST + LVWT + LVEDD)^3 - (LVEDD)^3] \times 1.05$ and left ventricular mass index was calculated as left ventricular mass divided by body surface area. Electrocardiograms and echocardiograms were performed every three months throughout the 18 month study.

Table 1. Study Plan.

	Diuretic Phase > 2 wks	Entry	Titration Phase 6 wks	Maintenance Phase 64 wks					
				3 mth	3 mth	3 mth	3 mth	3 mth	3 mth
Week	(−2) (−1)	0	1 2 3 4 5 6	19	32	45	58	60	72
Echo/ECG	X	X	X	X	X	X	X	X	X

Results

Of the 19 patients, 11 were categorized as "responders" and eight were "non-responders". The mean control and final blood pressure responses of both groups are shown in Table 2. Responders' mean blood pressures dropped from 19.1/15.8 mmHg compared with an even more brisk response, antihypertensive effect in the non-responders, 41.7/22.1 mmHg (Table 3). The mean dose of Combipres utilized in both responders and non-responder populations was virtually identical, 0.56 mg of clonidine/day versus 0.53 mg of clonidine/day. Left ventricular mass in the responders was diminished 45.10 g after 18 months of therapy. On the other hand, left ventricular mass increased 29.8 g among the eight non-responders. Septal thickness was diminished among both the 11 responders and eight non-responders (Table 4). Left ventricular posterior wall thickness was diminished among the responders (by 0.5 cm) and was slightly increased among the non-responders (by 0.3 cm). End-diastolic diameter was reduced among the responders as the left ventricular mass and left ventricular mass index; however each of these three parameters was increased among the non-responders.

---

* LVEDD = left ventricular end-diastolic diameter; LVWT = left ventricular wall thickness; T = posterior wall thickness; S = septal thickness.

Table 2. Blood Pressure (mmHg) Responses.

	11 Responders			
	Supine		Erect	
	Control	Final	Control	Final
Systolic	157.7	138.6	153.6	140.4
Diastolic	98.7	82.9	103.6	92.9
	8 Non-responders			
	Supine		Erect	
	Control	Final	Control	Final
Systolic	173.1	131.4	175.0	148.0
Diastolic	105.1	83.0	112.6	98.6

Table 3. Blood Pressure and Left Ventricular Mass Changes from Baseline.

	Supine BP Changes from baseline	Change in LVM from baseline	Mean dose of clonidine
11 Responders	Systolic 19.1 Diastolic 15.8	−45.10 g	0.56 mg
8 Non-responders	Systolic 41.7 Diastolic 22.148	+29.8 g	0.53 mg

Table 4. Left Ventricular Changes.

	11 Responders	
	Baseline	18 months
Septal thickness (cm)	1.45	1.37
Left ventricular posterior wall (cm)	1.43	1.38
End diastolic diameter (cm)	4.68	4.47
Left ventricular mass (g)	350.1	304.9
Left ventricular mass index (g/m²)	189.7	164.8
	8 Non-responders	
	Baseline	18 months
Septal thickness (cm)	1.53	1.47
Left ventricular posterior wall (cm)	1.37	1.40
End diastolic diameter (cm)	4.30	4.61
Left ventricular mass (g)	308.8	338.6
Left ventricular mass index (g/m²)	160.8	176.3

Utilizing the usual voltage criteria for electrocardiographic evidence of LVH (RVI + SV5 or 6), no consistent patterns were noted among either the responders or non-responders.

Discussion

The aetiology of cardiomegaly and more specifically of LVH is diverse. Viral infections, congenital heart disease, valvular heart disease, coronary artery disease, rheumatic heart disease, auto-immune deficiences, alcoholism, metabolic diseases, endocrine diseases, as well as systemic hypertension are well established causes. Several other factors such as age, race, obesity, hyperadrenergic stages, highly-conditioned athletes, high renin levels, systolic hypertension, and the male sex, all appear to be correlated with an increased incidence of LVH. It is not surprising then to learn from other therapeutic attempts to reverse LVH and to learn, too, from our own results, that not every hypertensive patient who has his hypertension adequately controlled (by drugs such as α_2-agonists, converting enzyme inhibitors, and β-blockers) will experience reversal or regression of his LVH. Concentric hypertrophy, eccentric hypertrophy, and predominantly septal hypertrophy have each been associated with untreated hypertension. But the aetiology of these various forms of ventricular enlargement is not elucidated.

Casual office blood pressures may not accurately reflect 24-hour blood pressures or indeed the "stress" pressures emphasised by Devereux et al. (1983).

In analysing our data (Table 5), it was evident that the mean age of the non-responders was 59.2 years (2.1 years older than the responders), their mean body weight was 184.5 lb (versus 176.8 lb in the responders), their duration of hypertension was less (10.6 years versus 16.4 years for the responders), and six out of eight (75%) of the non-responders were females versus 64% (seven out of 11) responders being females. It is possible, therefore, that this slight preponderance of females, a slightly older age group, and the slightly greater mean body weight, and perhaps the shorter duration of pre-existing hypertension, all contributed to the inability of the non-responders to reduce left ventricular mass. The reduction in size of the interventricular septal thickness was virtually identical in both the responder and non-responder groups. Much of the recent literature indicates that the severity of the systolic hypertension is related to the degree of septal hypertrophy, and reduction of systolic hypertension is generally associated with a good response of this particular parameter. This was so in our study where non-responders had higher systolic pressures initially (158 vs. 173 mmHg).

Significant reductions in LVM, LVMI, posterior wall thickness and interventricular septal thickness were evident as early as three months in most of the responders.

Surely one of the most critical potential variables in monitoring changes in LVH is dependent on the quality, i.e., the precision as well as the accuracy of the echocardiographic measurements. Early on in our study, we deliberately disguised five of our patients

Table 5. Demographic Data.

	Responders	Non-Responders
Total number of patients	11	8
Sex	7 Female	6 Female
	4 Male	2 Male
Average age	57.7	59.2
Average body weight	176.8 lb	184.5 lb
Average duration of hypertension	16.4 years	10.6 years

and obtained three separate echoes on each of them using pseudonyms, as well as physical disguise. The precision, i.e., reproducibility of the various echo measurements, was excellent. In addition to this, we coded and randomised all the echocardiograms and had them read in a blind fashion by a cardiologist at our university hospital who was completely ignorant about our study protocol. We therefore feel relatively assured that the echo measurements reported here are reliable.

Conclusions

Clonidine given at doses of approximately 0.6 mg daily together with chlorthalidone given at a total daily dose of approximately 90 mg (i.e., six tablets/day of Combipres) significantly reduced left ventricular hypertrophy in 11 out of 18 hypertensive patients (61%) with severe left ventricular hypertrophy. Left ventricular mass, left ventricular mass index, end-diastolic diameter, septal thickness, and left ventricular posterior wall diameter all diminished significantly, beginning at three months and continuing through 18 months of the study. There was no correlation whatsoever between the successful reduction of blood pressure and the reversal of left ventricular hypertrophy.

Since left ventricular hypertrophy is not exclusively due to sustained arterial hypertension, not all hypertensive patients with LVH can be expected to respond to effective drugs such as clonidine. Although concurrent diuretics were used and are known to fail to reduce (or even to enhance) LVH, the combination of the α_2-agonist, clonidine, with the diuretic, chlorthalidone, successfully reduced LVH in most patients.

Reference

1. Devereux RB, Pickering TG, Laragh J, et al (1983) Left ventricular hypertrophy in patients with hypertension of blood pressure response to regular recurring stress. Circulation 68 (3): 470–476

Authors' address:
F. Gilbert McMahon, M.D.
Department of Medicine
Tulane University School of Medicine
The Clinical Research Center
New Orleans, Louisiana 70112
U.S.A.

Pharmacodynamics and Pharmacokinetics of Oral and Transdermal Clonidine in Chronic Renal Insufficiency

David T. Lowenthal, Steven D. Saris, Bonita Falkner, R. Stephen Porter, Alan Haratz, Jeffrey Packer, Carol Bies, and Kathleen Conry

Introduction

Use of the skin as a means for drug delivery, especially transdermal application of nitroglycerine, has been receiving increasing attention in the area of cardiovascular medicine (Adkinson 1977; Karsh et al. 1978; Hansen et al. 1979; Müller et al. 1982; Colfer et al. 1982; Olivari and Cohn 1983). Although some controversy exists now about bioavailability and effectiveness, it still remains a viable alternative to sublingual and oral administration. Two antihypertensive drugs have been studied by means of application to the skin. Preliminary data on the transdermal application of timolol has shown that it is effective in blunting the exercise response in normals (Lowenthal et al. unpublished). Further studies on its effectiveness as an antihypertensive when applied transdermally are being initiated.

The application of transdermal clonidine (clonidine-TTS) in the treatment of hypertension (Weber et al. 1984; Mroczek 1983) has been a major breakthrough for drug delivery in the treatment of hypertension both in the uncomplicated and in the complicated phases. It is effective in the management of mild to moderate rises in blood pressure, well tolerated, with minimal skin irritation, and the side-effects of xerostomia and drowsiness are less intense.

Chronic renal failure is often associated with hypertension and other abnormalities involving the endocrine, cardiac, nervous and musculoskeletal system; thus, renal insufficiency is truly a systemic process. The skin, nails and mucous membranes are not spared in this regard. The purpose of this study was to examine the effectiveness of clonidine-TTS in patients with different degrees of renal impairment and to compare the preliminary results with data obtained with oral clonidine in patients with impaired renal function, juveniles with hypertension and the elderly with and without parenchymal renal disease.

Patients and Methods

The pharmacodynamic effects of oral and transdermal clonidine were studied in eight hypertensive patients (four men and four women, age range 18–65), six whose creatinine

---

Likoff Cardiovascular Institute and the Department of Pediatrics and Medicine, Hahnemann University, Philadelphia, Pennsylvania, U.S.A.

clearance was between 6 ml/min and 50 ml/min and two whose renal function was absent and who were maintained on haemodialysis three times weekly. All of the patients had long-standing primary hypertension and were being treated with various antihypertensive medications before the start of the study. All antihypertensive drugs were gradually withdrawn over a two-week period. Following this washout phase, each of the patients was given clonidine 0.1 mg twice daily with frusemide or hydrochlorothiazide in a dosage necessary to maintain an oedema-free state. Clonidine was increased up to 0.3 mg twice daily in order to obtain a diastolic blood pressure of less than 95 mmHg in the sitting position. Once the endpoint for the diastolic pressure was reached the patient was then switched to a comparable patch whose dosage approximated that maximum dosage achieved with the oral preparation.

Blood for clonidine analysis was obtained at the end of the oral clonidine period in the morning just before the usual morning dosage (trough level) and two hours after this dosage (peak level). Additional plasma clonidine samples were obtained at the end of the titration with the clonidine patch phase of the study.

Clonidine was assayed by RIA methodology (Arndts et al. 1981; Arndts et al. 1983). This method detects pure clonidine and does not quantify any of the questionably active metabolites.

In a previous study, blood was drawn for clonidine concentration once steady-state dosing had been achieved. Simultaneously blood pressure and heart rate recordings were monitored in hypertensive adolescents, and in adults of different ages and with various degrees of renal impairment.

All of the patients with advanced renal disease were on ferrous sulphate, multivitamins, aluminium hydroxide gel or capsules, and folic acid.

Results

The salient pharmacodynamic features comparing the oral and TTS data are summarised in Table 1 and Figures 1 and 2. Once the patients were switched to clonidine-TTS, blood pressure remained controlled compared to the end of the oral clonidine titration period; the dosage was equivalent to that required with the oral administration and the adverse effects of dryness of the mouth and sedation were present, but better tolerated. The dosage of frusemide in five patients ranged from 40–160 mg daily and that of hydrochlorothiazide was 50 mg in one patient. There was no evidence of erythema or blister formation within the area of patch application. When compared to the mean heart rate on oral dosage, i.e. 76, there was a slight but insignificant reduction in heart rate, i.e. 72, with the application of clonidine-TTS.

In patients whose creatinine clearance was greater than 5 ml/min and less than 50 ml/min the range of plasma clonidine concentrations following the titration of the oral dose was 0.56–6.6 ng/ml and that at the stable dose on patch, 1.22–4.1 ng/ml. The two dialysis maintained patients had oral and transdermal plasma clonidine concentrations of 5.75–11.4 and 4.93–11.0 ng/ml respectively (Fig. 3).

Because the adolescent and geriatric hypertensive populations represent two groups which may have compromised renal function leading to clonidine accumulation, steady-state plasma clonidine concentrations were determined in these groups after dose titration to the maximum antihypertensive effect. The results are summarized in Table 2: in chil-

Table 1. Pharmacodynamic Responses to Oral Clonidine and Clonidine-TTS.

	Mean Daily Clonidine Dose (mg)	Supine BP	Standing BP	HR Supine
Pre-clonidine Titration	–	155/101	149/105	79
End of Clonidine Titration	0.39 mg[e]	131/94[a]	121/91[c]	76[e]
4 weeks of TTS	= # 2 patch 0.49 mg[e]	135/91[b]	131/91[d]	72[e]

[a] $p < 0.01$; [b] $p < .02$; [c] $p < .01$; [d] $p < .05$; [e] N.S.

Fig. 1. Supine systolic and diastolic blood pressure pretreatment, after oral clonidine titration and during TTS therapy.

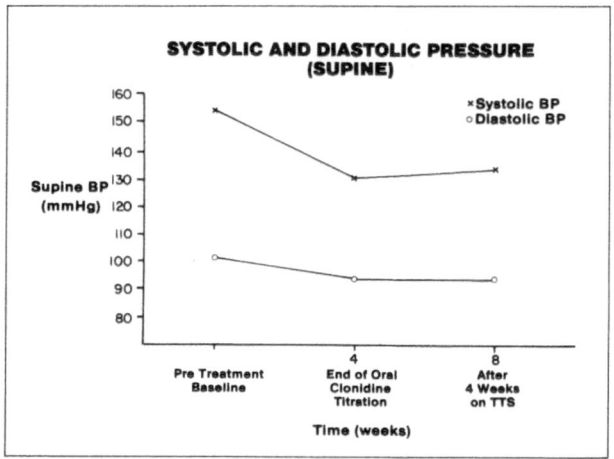

Fig. 2. Standing systolic and diastolic blood pressure pretreatment, after oral clonidine titration and during TTS therapy.

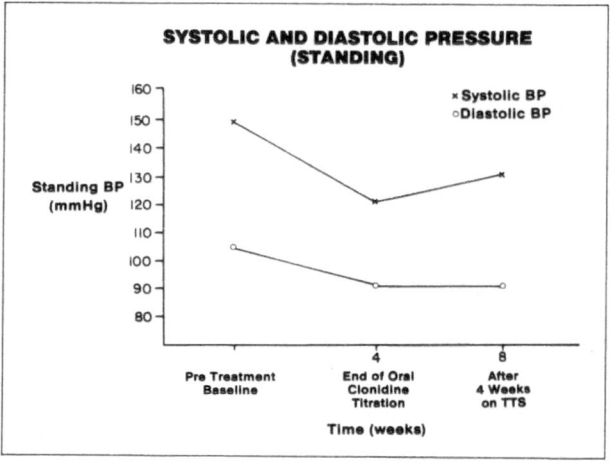

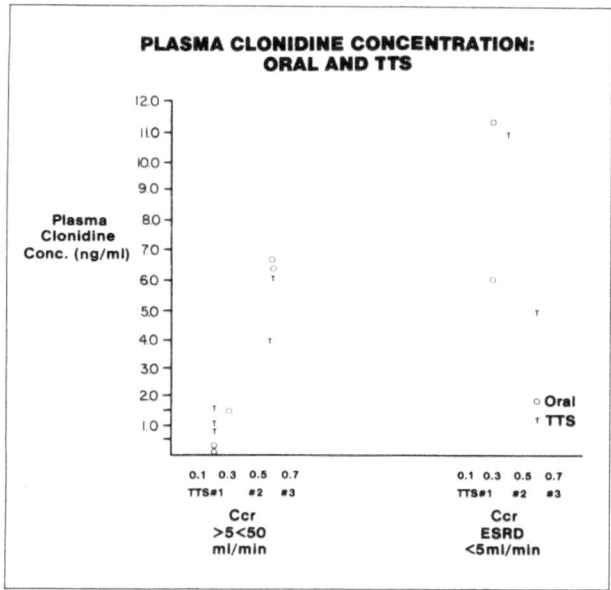

Fig. 3. Plasma clonidine concentrations at peak of oral clonidine and during stable TTS dosage according to renal function.

dren 11–18 years old, requiring 0.2 mg/day, steady-state plasma concentrations were 0.38 ± 0.17 ng/ml. In those adolescents requiring 0.4 mg per day, plasma concentration was 1.22 ng/ml. Adolescents with poor blood pressure control who were also found to be non-compliant to drug therapy had plasma clonidine concentrations less than 0.1 ng/ml. In young normotensive adults on 0.2 mg/day, a mean plasma clonidine concentration of 0.7 ng/ml was achieved. In adults over 40 years old, steady-state plasma concentration ranged from 0.1 to 3.4 ng/ml (0.2–0.8 mg oral clonidine per day) with satisfactory blood pressure control. These data contrast with the higher plasma clonidine concentrations seen in dialysis patients, regardless of age. One patient with a serum creatinine of 2 mg/dl had a clonidine concentration of 2.8 ng/ml and a diastolic pressure of 116 mmHg and another with ESRD had a clonidine value of 3.0 ng/ml with a diastolic pressure of 120 mmHg. Most patients whose clonidine concentrations were beyond the "therapeutic window" of 0.8–2.0 ng/ml had diastolic pressures less than 90 mmHg (Table 2).

Discussion

The results of this study indicate that clonidine taken orally and then applied transdermally reduces blood pressure and maintains the reduction in blood pressure achieved at the maximum oral dosage. The patients tolerated the patch with no greater incidence of adverse effects than that which had been experienced while taking the oral preparation. Furthermore, drowsiness and dry mouth were no more apparent in those patients with very high plasma clonidine concentrations than those with lower clonidine concentrations.

The high plasma clonidine concentrations in the setting of impaired renal function were associated in general with control of blood pressure (Tables 1 and 2, Fig. 3). Whether this

89

Table 2. Plasma Concentrations of Clonidine Required to Maintain Diastolic Pressure < 90 mmHg.

Adolescents Ages 11–18		Normotensive Adults with Normal Renal Function < 40 years old		Adults > 40 years with Normal Renal Function		
Dose (mg/day)	Conc (ng/ml)	Dose (mg/day)	Conc (ng/ml)	Dose (mg/day)	Conc (ng/ml)	Age
0.2	0.38 ± 0.17	0.2	0.57 ± 12	<0.2	1.4	80
n = 11		n = 6			1.9	71
0.4	1.22 ± 0.41			0.2–0.8	0.1	42
n = 4					0.5	68
					3.0	65
				>0.8	3.4	45

Uncontrolled BP	Adults < 40 Years with End Stage Renal Disease (ESRD)		Adults > 40 Years with Abnormal Renal Function		
Conc < 0.1	Dose (mg/day)	Conc (ng/ml)	Dose (mg/day)	Conc (ng/ml)	Age
	<0.2	3.0*	<0.2	0.5	42
n = 6				2.1	60
	0.2–0.6	6.1		3.1	45
		7.2	0.2–0.8	2.8	68**
				7.5	45
			0.9	9.0	52

* DBP = 120; ** Serum creatinine 2.0 mg/dl and DBP = 116, all others have ESRD.

phenomenon of high concentrations and control of systemic arterial blood pressure in this patient population may be related to altered (decreased) peripheral α-receptor response and inability to develop vasoconstriction has yet to be ascertained. There is precedent for autonomic insufficiency and altered tissue sensitivity in ESRD (Lowenthal and Reidenberg 1972; Pickering et al. 1972; Lazarus et al. 1973). In the case of clonidine this may include a decrease in response at both α_1 and α_2 peripheral loci.

Clonidine is almost completely absorbed and distributed throughout the body. Approximately 30% is metabolised in the liver and the remaining 70% with its questionably active metabolites are excreted principally by the kidneys (Lowenthal 1980). The metabolites of clonidine are alkaline, neutral, and acidic conjugates and play a minor rôle in man. The pharmacokinetics may be described by a first-order, two-compartment open model with an elimination half-life in normals ranging from 5–13 hours. Normally there is no accumulation of clonidine with chronic administration (Keranen et al. 1978). However, the elimination half-life is prolonged in patients with renal insufficiency and no replacement of clonidine is necessary after dialysis (Lowenthal et al. 1983). There seems to be a close correlation between plasma clonidine concentration, side-effects and pharmacodynamic response.

Since chronic renal insufficiency is a systemic disease with the latter being also represented in the skin, it is uncertain whether transdermal application of drugs is subtherapeutic, effective, or associated with enhanced absorption in patients with renal insufficiency. Skin pigmentation occurs due to urochrome accumulation. Calcification of the skin can likewise occur as a consequence of secondary hyperparathyroidism. The pigmentation is not known to interfere with drug absorption but calcification certainly can prevent drug absorption. Progressive systemic sclerosis (scleroderma), polyarteritis nodosa and systemic lupus erythematosus are several of the dermal-renal entities which can cause such a degree of subcutaneous disease as to prevent adequate drug absorption. None of the patients in this study had his her renal insufficiency on the basis of collagen vascular disease and none had overt manifestations of the dermal involvement secondary to hyperparathyroidism. In addition, none of them had pruritis which would cause excoriation of the skin and possibly enhance drug absorption (Groth et al. 1983). Although drug delivery transdermally has not been adequately studied in patients with chronic renal insufficiency with regards to comparative bioavailability between dermal and enteral absorption, this study provides some information about the close relationship between oral and transdermal clonidine pharmacodynamic response. It appears that the dosage delivered by the patch was equivalent to that dosage reached maximally during the oral titration phase of the study. However, the transdermal plasma clonidine concentrations appear slightly lower than those with oral dosing. The equal reduction in blood pressure may represent better compliance and less fluctuation in plasma-pressure variations with patch usage.

In conclusion, clonidine-TTS is an effective and safe alternative to oral clonidine in the management of hypertension associated with renal insufficiency.

Acknowledgement

The authors wish to thank Darla Chase for her secretarial assistance and Joseph Wasilnak for his help in the performance of this study.

References

1. Adkinson HW (1977) Standardised regimen for applying nitroglycerine ointment. Am J Cardiol 40: 143
2. Arndts D, Doevendans J, Kirsten R, Heintz B (1983) New aspects of the pharmacokinetics and pharmacodynamics of clonidine in man. Eur J Clin Pharmacol 24: 21–30
3. Arndts D, Stahle H, Forster HJ (1983) Development of an RIA for clonidine and its comparison with reference methods. J Pharmacol Methods 6: 295–307
4. Colfer H, Stetson P, Lucchesi BR, Wagner J, Pitt B (1982) The nitroglycerine polymer get matrix system: a new method for administering nitroglycerine evaluated with plasma nitroglycerine level. J Cardiovas Pharmacol 4: 521–525
5. Davies DS, Wing LMH, Reid JL, Neill E, Tippitt P, Dollery CT (1977) Pharmacokinetics and concentration effect relationships of intravenous and oral clonidine. Clin Pharmacol Therap 21: 593–601
6. Dollery CT, Davies DS, Draffan GH, Dargie HJ, Dean CR, Reid JL (1976) Clinical pharmacology and pharmacokinetics of clonidine. Clin Pharmacol Therap 19: 11–17
7. Groth H, Vetter H, Knuesel J, Vetter W, McMahon FG, Weber MA (1983) Allergic skin reactions to transdermal clonidine. Lancet 2: 850–851
8. Hansen MS, Woods SL, Willis RE (1979) Relative effectiveness of nitroglycerine ointment according to site of application. Heart & Lung 8: 716–720
9. Karsh, DL, Umbach RE, Cohen LS, Langau RA (1978) Prolonged benefit of nitroglycerine ointment on exercise tolerance in patients with angina pectoris. Am Heart J 96: 587–595

10. Keranen A, Nykanen S, Taskinen J (1978) Pharmacokinetics and side effects of clonidine. Eur J Clin Pharmacol 13: 97–101
11. Lazarus JM, Hampers Cl, Lowrie EG, Merrill JP (1973) Baroreceptor activity in normotensive and hypertensive uremic patients. Circ 47: 1015–1021
12. Lowenthal DT (1980) Pharmacokinetics of clonidine. J Cardiovas Pharmacol 2 (Suppl 1): s29–s37
13. Lowenthal DT, Affrime MB, Meyer A, Kim K, Falkner B, Shariff K (1983) Pharmacokinetics and pharmacodynamics of clonidine in varying states of renal function. Chest 83s: 386s–390s
14. Lowenthal DT, Reidenberg MM (1972) The heart rate response to atropine in uremic patients, obese subjects before and during fasting and patients with other chronic illnesses. Proceedings Society Experimental Biology Medicine 139: 390–393
15. Mroczek WJ (1983) Preliminary evaluation of transdermal clonidine administration in hypertensive patients receiving a diuretic. In: Catapres: Pathways in the Development of a Pharmaceutical, Bock KD (Ed), Editio Cantor Aulendorf F.R.G. p 126–132
16 Müller P, Imhof PR, Burkart F, Chu LC, Gerordin A (1982) Human pharmacological studies of a new transdermal system containing nitroglycerine. Eur J Clin Pharmacol 22: 473–480
17. Olivari MT, Cohn JN (1983) Cutaneous administration of nitroglycerine: a review. Pharmacotherapy 3: 149–157
18. Pickering TG, Gribbin B, Oliver DO (1972) Baroreflex sensitivity in patients on long-term hemodialysis. Clin Sci 43: 645–657
19. Weber MA, Drayer JIM, Brewer DD, Lipson JL (1984) Transdermal continuous antihypertensive therapy. Lancet 1: 9–11

Authors' address:
David T. Lowenthal, M.D.
Likoff Cardiovascular Institut
Department of Pediatrics and Medicine
Hahnemann University
Philadelphia, Pennsylvania 19102
U.S.A.

A Multicenter Study on the Use of Transdermal Clonidine in Patients with Essential Hypertension

Jan I. M. Drayer, Michael A. Weber, and Deborah D. Brewer

Introduction

Non-diuretic antihypertensive agents now are frequently used in the treatment of patients with mild essential hypertension (Campese 1980; Mroczek 1983). In these patients, blood pressure is often controlled using oral therapy with a single agent. Recently, a new delivery system for monotherapy with the centrally-acting sympatholytic agent clonidine has become available. In this study, we describe the results of a multicenter study using an adhesive skin device containing clonidine (Catapres-TTS). The results indicate that treatment with a transdermal delivery system for clonidine is effective and well tolerated in patients with mild hypertension.

Methods

The study was carried out at five institutions. All patients who participated in the study (n = 101) had mild essential hypertension with seated diastolic blood pressures between 91 and 104 mmHg. Secondary causes of hypertension were excluded using standard clinical and laboratory methods. Patients with overt heart disease, chronic lung disease, kidney disease or liver disease, or diabetes mellitus were excluded from entry into the study. All patients signed informed consents as approved by the institutional review board of the participating institutions.

Patients who complied with the entry criteria of the study were then treated using a transdermal delivery system for clonidine. The transdermal delivery system did not contain active medication during the placebo phase of the study. At the end of the placebo period, patients were given a delivery system containing clonidine. This system is made to deliver approximately 0.1 mg of clonidine daily for a one-week period. The number of systems given to each patient was increased at weekly intervals until control of blood pressure was achieved. Control of blood pressure was defined as a fall in seated diastolic blood pressure of at least 10 mmHg or a fall in diastolic blood pressure to less than 90 mmHg. Treatment was continued at the end of the titration period during a three-month maintenance phase.

Blood pressure was measured with a standard mercury sphygmomanometer. Blood samples were obtained at the end of the placebo period and at the end of the maintenance

Section of Clinical Pharmacology and Hypertension, Veterans Administration Medical Center, Long Beach, California, and the University of California, Irvine, California, U.S.A.

93

phase. Routine analysis of serum creatinine, uric acid, and serum electrolytes was performed. Statistical analysis was done using the paired Student's t-test. Values are expressed as mean ± SEM.

Results

There were 69 patients who completed the titration period and 67 of these patients completed the maintenance phase without protocol violations. Of the 69 patients 28 were white and 41 were black, 46 patients were male and 23 were female. At the end of the titration period, blood pressure was controlled, as defined for this protocol, in 17 patients with one delivery system, in 28 patients with two systems and in nine patients using three systems. The responses in systolic and diastolic blood pressure are depicted in Figures 1 and 2.

Figure 1 shows that 83% of patients reached systolic blood pressures of less than 150 mmHg and that 71% of patients reached diastolic blood pressures equal to or less than 90 mmHg at the end of the titration period. The percentages were 76% and 75%, respectively, at the end of the maintenance period.

Blood pressure was 146 ± 18 (SD) over 96 ± 4 mmHg at the end of the placebo period, 137 ± 17 over 88 ± 8 mmHg at the end of the titration period and 138 ± 20 over 87 ± 6 mmHg at the end of the maintenance period. The decreases in blood pressure were highly significant ($p < 0.01$ or better).

Changes in serum potassium, creatinine, uric acid, glucose, cholesterol, high density lipoproteins and triglycerides observed during treatment with transdermal clonidine were not significant.

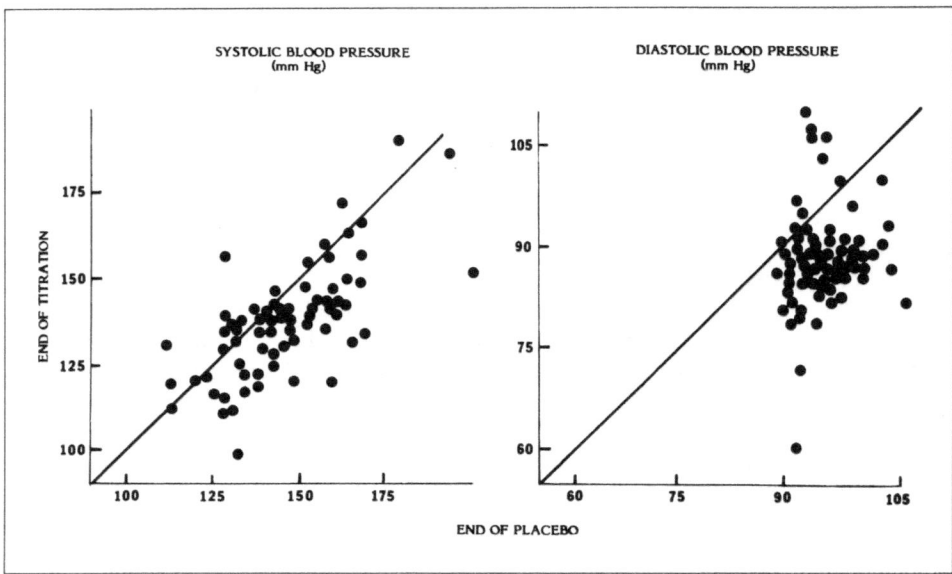

Fig. 1. The effect of transdermally administered clonidine on systolic and diastolic blood pressure at the end of the titration period.

94

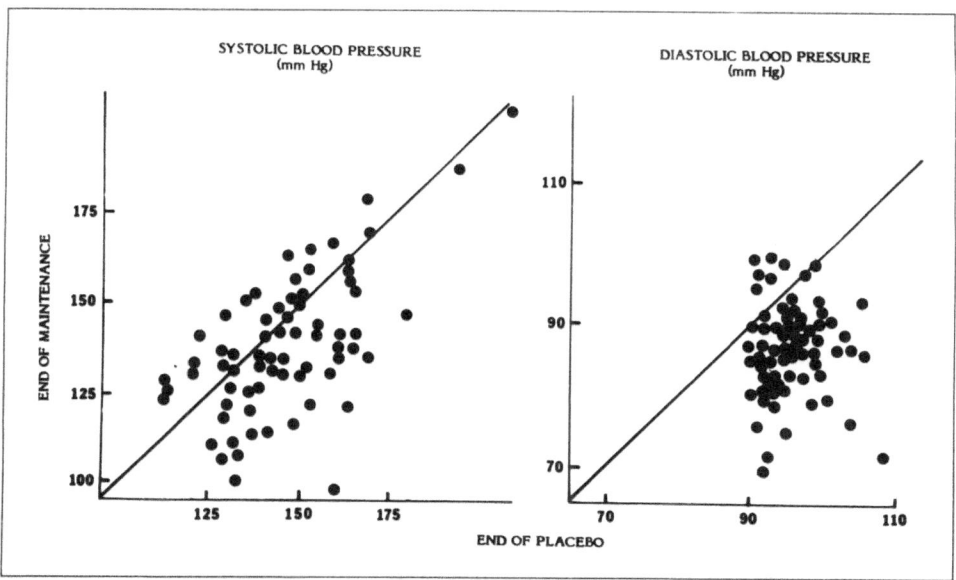

Fig. 2. The effect of transdermally administered clonidine on systolic blood pressure at the end of the maintenance period.

Mild side-effects were observed in some patients during treatment with transdermal clonidine. Most side-effects occurred only once during the study. Dry mouth was reported in 31% of the patients, a slight drowsiness was reported in 16%. Eight patients (9%) reported definite dermatological responses to the use of the transdermal system. The most commonly observed reaction consisted of erythema with or without pruritis. All changes reversed shortly after removal of the patch.

Discussion

In this paper we reviewed the clinical experiences with transdermally-administered clonidine in 85 patients with mild essential hypertension. The results reveal that transdermal delivery of small doses of this potent antihypertensive agent successfully controls blood pressure in over 50% of patients. Others have shown that transdermal clonidine is as effective as oral clonidine when given to patients with diuretic resistant hypertension (Popli 1983).

It was shown that blood pressure is controlled during the use of the transdermal application of clonidine with a smaller dose of clonidine. Therefore, blood levels of clonidine are less during transdermal application of clonidine than during oral administration of this drug (Popki 1983; Weber and Drayer 1984; Weber et al. 1984). Similarly, drug levels observed in a subset of patients included in this multicenter study revealed low blood levels of clonidine (Weber et al. 1978).

We have reported that after replacement of the active drug delivery system by a placebo, blood pressure gradually returns to the pretreatment level (Weber et al. 1978). The ab-

95

sence of rebound phenomena might be a reflection of the low drug levels of clonidine found in our patients.

Most patients considered the once-weekly transdermal application of drug more convenient than oral administration of drugs. However, the effect of long-term application of drug delivery systems on the skin remains to be solved. In our study we reported only mild skin reactions such as erythema or pruritus. However, others have reported skin reactions in a significant number of cases. The importance of these findings as well as the solution to this problem has been discussed extensively elsewhere in this book.

The transdermal application of clonidine seems to be an effective new tool in the treatment of patients with mild hypertension. The drug can be applied as monotherapy or in combination with low doses of other drugs, such as diuretics or vasodilators, given orally. The relative absence of significant side-effects will further add to the patient compliance with antihypertensive therapy.

Acknowledgement

The multicenter study was performed at five centres in the United States including the University of Texas Health Science Center in Dallas (Dr. Kirk), the Clinical Research Center in New Orleans (Dr. McMahon), and Veterans Administration Medical Centers in Cleveland (Dr. Shah), Boston (Dr. Hamburger) and Long Beach (Drs. Drayer and Weber).

References

1. Campese VM, Romoff M, Telfer N et al (1980) Role of sympathetic nerve inhibition and body sodium-volume state in the antihypertensive action of clonidine in essential hypertension. Kidney Int 18: 351–357
2. Mroczek WJ (1983) Preliminary evaluation of transdermal clonidine administration in hypertensive patients receiving a diuretic. In: Bock KD (ed.) Catapresan. Editio Cantor, Aulendorf, p 126–132
3. Popli S, Stroka G, Ing TS, Daugirdas JT, Norusis MJ, Hano JE, Gandhi VC (1983) Transdermal clonidine for hypertensive patients. Clin Ther 5: 624–628
4. Weber MA, Drayer JIM (1984) Clinical experience with rate controlled delivery of antihypertensive therapy by a transdermal system. Am Heart J (in press)
5. Weber MA, Drayer JIM, Brewer DD, Lipson JL (1984) Transdermal continuous antihypertensive therapy. Lancet 1: 9–11
6. Weber MA, Drayer JIM, Laragh JH (1978) The effects of clonidine and propranolol, separately and in combination, on blood pressure and plasma renin activity in essential hypertension. J Clin Pharmacol 18: 233–240

Authors' address:
Jan I. M. Drayer, M.D.
Hypertension Center
Veterans Administration Medical Center
5901 East Seventh Street
Long Beach, California 90822
U.S.A.

Antihypertensive Action of Catapres-TTS

P. Balansard[1], T. Danays[2], A. Baralla[1], Y. Frances[3], and Ph. Sans[1]

Introduction

Clonidine is a centrally acting agent which is widely used as antihypertensive monotherapy in the elderly. A transdermal therapeutic system containing sufficient clonidine to maintain a rate-controlled release and effective plasma levels of the drug for seven days has been set up (Catapres-TTS) (Shaw et al. 1983; Arndts 1984). This new route of administration is effective in the treatment of mild and moderate essential hypertension (Popli et al. 1983; Weber et al. 1984). Long-term patient compliance and side-effects have to be evaluated. We have studied the blood pressure variations during different designs of administration of transdermal clonidine.

Methods

The antihypertensive action of Catapres-TTS was studied using blood pressure profiles (P) (automatic recording of blood pressure every quarter of an hour for twelve hours 8.00 h to 20.00 h with DINAMAP 845 apparatus). Four parameters were measured: mean blood pressure (MBP), systolic blood pressure (SBP), diastolic blood pressure (DBP), heart rate (HR) (Fig. 1). Independent of the protocol used, the means of the various parameters were compared by Student's t-test. The difference was considered to be significant when $p < 0.05$. The patients selected for the study showed more than 20% of their blood pressure readings greater than 160/95 mmHg (Balansard et al. 1984). The study was fully explained to each patient.

Results

Five protocols were used:

1. TTS 1 followed by TTS 1 (15 patients) (Fig. 2)

Most of the hypertensive patients were elderly; 13 were older than 70 years and only two were younger than 60 years.

---

[1] Service de Cardiologie, Centre Hospitalier Général de Toulon, France,
[2] Laboratoires Boehringer Ingelheim, Reims Cedex, France and
[3] Service de Médecine Interne et des Urgences, Pr R. Luccioni, Hôpital Nord, Chemin des Bourrely, Marseille, France.

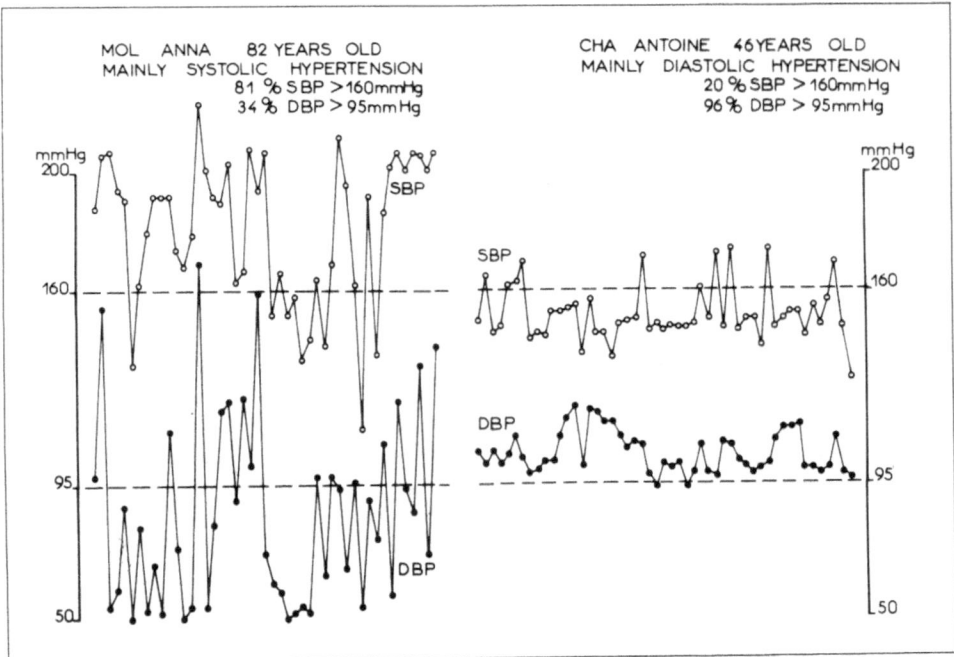

Fig. 1.

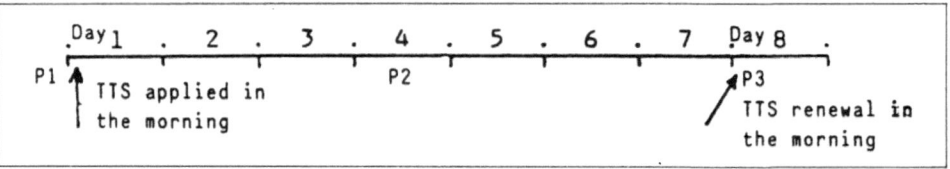

Fig. 2.

The antihypertensive action evaluated on the fourth day and on the eighth day.
Fourth day: There was a significant drop in three parameters (MBP, SBP, DBP) in six patients (40%) (Fig. 1), in two parameters (MBP, DBP) in one patient (6.7%) and in one parameter (SBP) in one patient (6.7%). TTS was ineffective in seven patients (46.7%). The percentage decrease in the mean blood pressure in those patients whose blood pressure dropped significantly in comparison with the control value was 14 ± 6.2% for MBP, 14.1 ± 5.9% for SBP and 16 ± 6.9% for DBP.

Eighth day: There was a significant decrease in three parameters in six patients (40%) (Fig. 3). There was a significant decrease on both the fourth and eighth day in only four patients (26.7%), in two parameters (SBP, DBP) in one patient (6.7%) and in one parameter (SBP) in two patients (13.3%). TTS was ineffective in five patients (on both the fourth and eighth day) and in one patient, TTS was effective on the fourth day but ineffective on the eighth day.

98

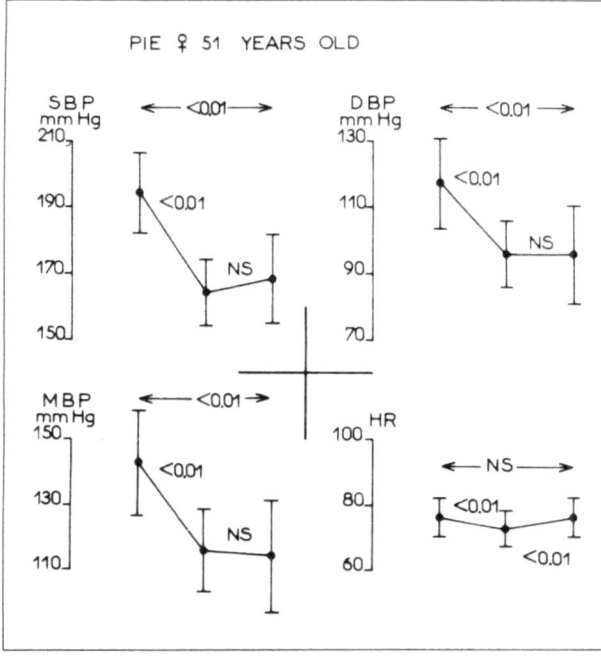

Fig. 3.

Action on heart rate

Fourth day: The heart rate had significantly decreased in eight patients (53.3%), was unchanged in six (40%) and had significantly increased in three (20%). In these last three patients, TTS did not have any antihypertensive action.

Eighth day: The heart rate had significantly decreased in 11 patients (73.3%) and was unchanged in four patients (26.7%).

Action on the variability of the blood pressure

This was evaluated by studying the means of the standard deviations and the mean maximum and minimum blood pressures in responders.

Table 1. Fourth day.

Standard deviations				
MBP:	21.9 ± 8.2	20.3 ± 8.3	NS	
SBP:	15.6 ± 3.4	16.1 ± 4.4	NS	
DBP:	22.0 ± 8.3	18.0 ± 8.6	NS	
Maximum pressure				
MBP:	182.8 ± 22.7	160.1 ± 23.8	t = 2.379	p < 0.05
SBP:	211.0 ± 18.3	194.3 ± 20.0	t = 2.584	p < 0.05
DBP:	164.5 ± 22.8	138.1 ± 26.4	t = 2.546	p < 0.05
	Minimum pressure			
MBP:	94.5 ± 11.5	79.6· ± 11.5	t = 9.313	p < 0.01
SBP:	134.5 ± 17.9	117.5· ± 25.2	NS	
DBP:	79.8 ± 10.8	64.4 ± 9.8	t = 7.942	p < 0.01

Eighth day: The results were identical. The mean of the minimum recording of SBP decreased significantly (p < 0.001). Thus, overall, TTS does not decrease the variability of blood pressure.

2. Changeover from 0.150 mg tablets to TTS 1 (five patients) (Fig. 4)

On the second day of recording under TTS, there was a significant fall in the three blood pressure parameters compared with the control values in all five patients. In two patients, the blood pressure did not fall significantly on the first day of treatment, suggesting that in some cases TTS has a delayed effect (Fig. 5).

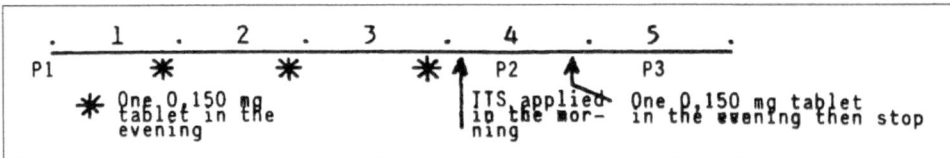

Fig. 4.

Fig. 5.

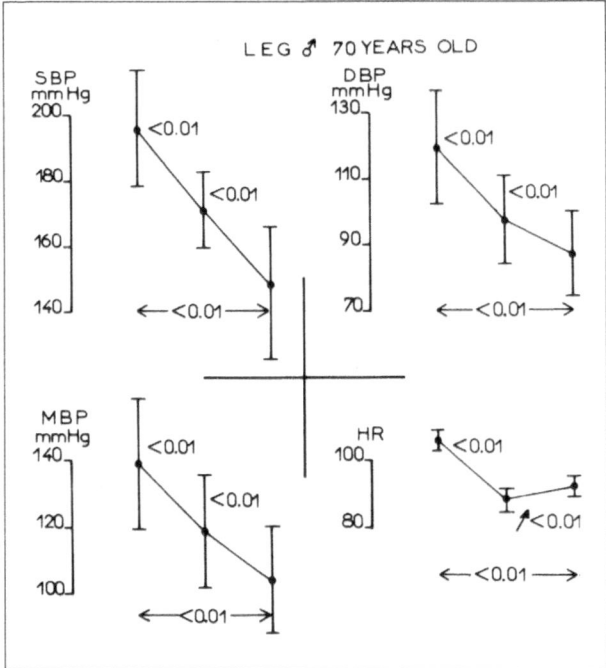

3. Withdrawal of TTS 1 (six patients) (Fig. 6)

In the two cases in which TTS was effective, there was no rise in blood pressure on the day following removal of the patch, which suggests that TTS may act for 48 hours (Fig. 7).

100

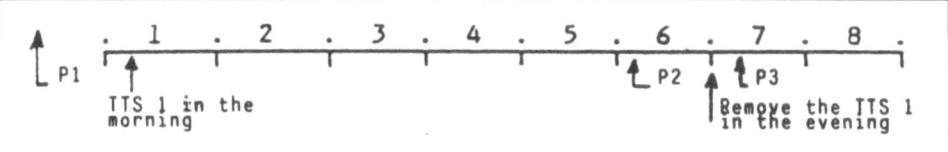

Fig. 6.

Fig. 7.

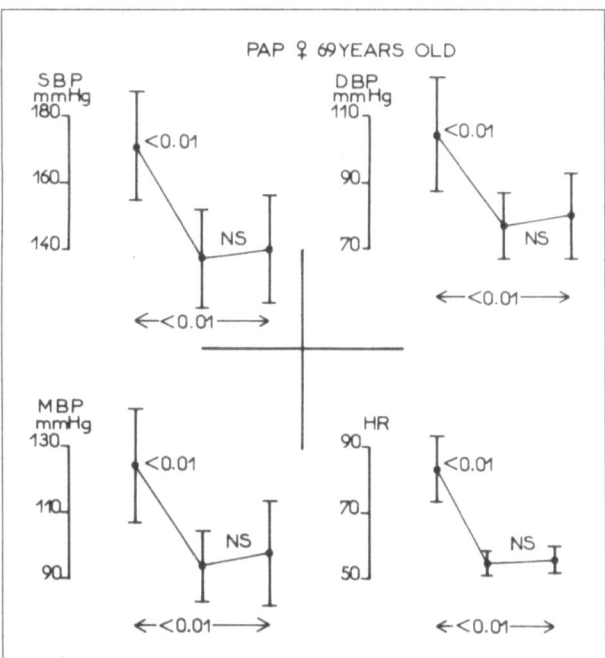

4. TTS 1 followed by TTS 2 (seven patients) (Fig. 8)

In seven cases in which TTS 1 was ineffective, it was replaced by TTS 2. On the seventh day of TTS 2 we recorded a significant decrease in the three blood pressure parameters in three patients (43%), in two parameters (MBP, SBP) in one patient (14%) and in one parameter (SBP or DBP) in two patients (28%). TTS was ineffective in one patient (Fig. 9).

5. Mid-term treatment

After an initial phase, the TTS was changed every seventh day. Readings were made every month on the seventh day after application of the fourth patch. The last recording was made after one month of treatment in one case, after two months of treatment in four cases, during the eighth month in one case and during the tenth month in two cases. TTS 1 was replaced by TTS 2 in three patients. In one patient, TTS was ineffective after one

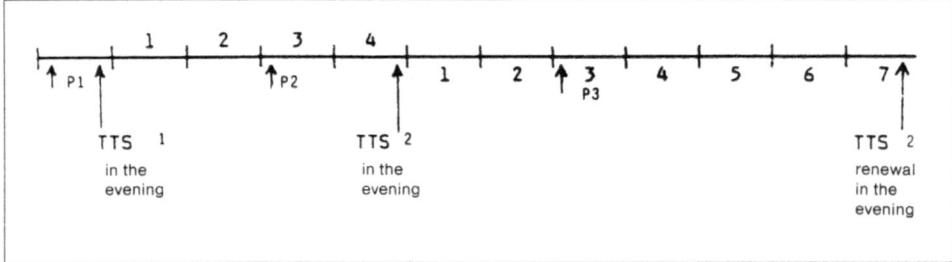

Fig. 8.

Fig. 9.

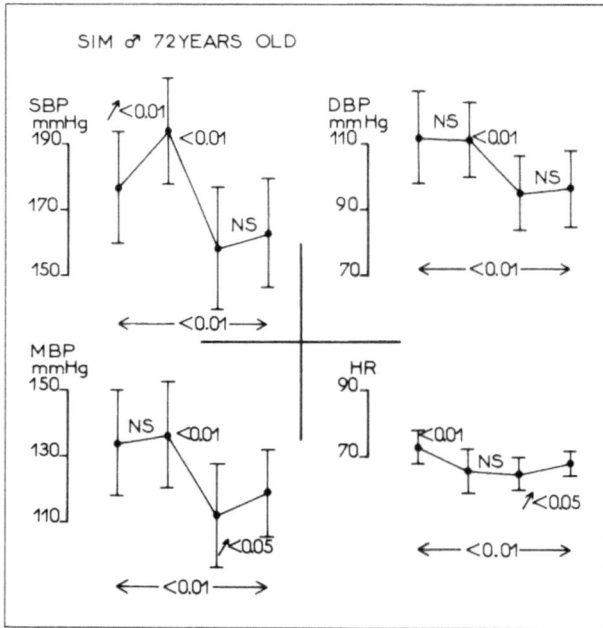

week of treatment and remained ineffective, with no change in the dose by the second month (Fig. 10).

6. Side-effects

TTS was stopped in two patients because of persistent pruriginous erythema (TTS 1 in one case and TTS 2 in the other). One patient, for whom the dose was increased to TTS 2 because of poor effectiveness, developed a dry mouth and the dose had to be decreased to TTS 1.

Conclusion

Short-term, TTS 1 is effective on the three parameters of blood pressure in 40% of cases. When this dose does not induce a partial or complete significant decrease in the blood pressure, increasing the dose to TTS 2 decreases the blood pressure parameters in 43%

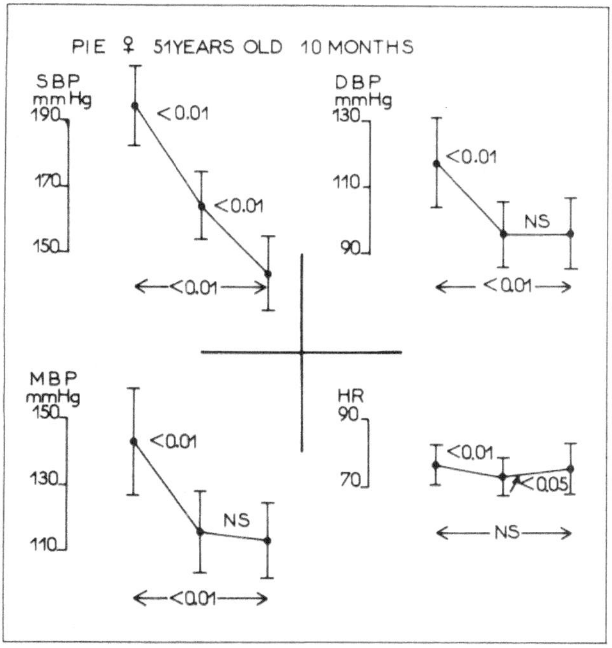

Fig. 10.

of cases. Overall therefore, TTS at either dose is effective in 66% of cases. Changing from the tablet form to TTS does not cause any significant rise in blood pressure. Withdrawal from TTS does not provoke any rebound phenomena. The intermediate-term study, with or without a change of dose, shows a continuing antihypertensive effect. The need to change the TTS only once a week makes the treatment very simple for the patient to follow.

References

1. Arndts D, Arndts K (1984) Pharmacokinetics and pharmacodynamics of transdermally administered clonidine. Eur J Clin Pharmacol 26: 79–85
2. Balansard P, Aubert P, Baralla A, Frances Y, Normand Ph, Camuzet JP, Sans Ph (1984) Relations entre clinique, paraclinique et profils tensionnels chez les hypertendus agés. Sem Hôp Paris 60: n°26 1865–1870
3. Popli S, Stroka G, Ing TS, Daugirdas JT, Norusis MJ, Hano JE, Gandhi VG (1983) Transdermal clonidine for hypertensive patients. Clin Ther 5: 624–626
4. Shaw JE, Enscore D, Chu L Clonidine rate – controlled system: technology and kinetics. In: Weber MA and Mathias CJ (Eds) Mild Hypertension. Proceedings of the International Titisee Workshop, October 13–15 1983. Steinkopff Verlag Darmstadt
5. Weber MA, Drayer JIM, Brewer DD, Lipson JL (1984) Transdermal continuous antihypertensive therapy. Lancet 1: 8363 9–11

Authors' address:
P. Balansard, M.D.
Service de Cardiologie
Centre Hospitalier Général de Toulon
1208 avenue Colonel Picot
83100 Toulon
France

Discussion

WEBER:

I should like to follow up on Dr. Kolloch's paper. I was interested in your comparison of clonidine with the β-blocker, metoprolol. I thought it was particularly important that you were able to achieve antihypertensive responses with clonidine given in oral doses of 0.0375 mg twice daily. This is obviously a lower dose than is customarily administered, and indicates that we may be using oral clonidine in excessive doses in many of our patients. It is certainly an attractive possibility that very low doses of the drug, with which there are only minimal side-effects, might be clinically effective. What sort of plasma concentrations are seen with this very low dosing of clonidine, and how do these levels compare with the concentrations achieved during transdermal treatment?

KOLLOCH:

We believe that the effectiveness of the low oral doses we have given to be comparable to the use of a standard small transdermal clonidine patch. The plasma clonidine concentrations during these two forms of treatment also appear to be very similar. I believe that the primary antihypertensive action of clonidine, which is suppression of sympathetic nervous activity, can be adequately achieved with these very low doses. I suspect that the use of higher doses produces other pharmacological actions, some of which are not necessary and may be associated with producing some of the side-effects that can cause problems for the patient.

WEBER:

I believe that the work done by Dr. Kolloch and some of his European colleagues has been very important in drawing attention to the potential efficacy of the very low oral doses of clonidine. Studies performed with transdermal clonidine have shown that it has similar efficacy to oral clonidine treatment even when it is administered at lower doses. Some of the crossover studies, in which oral clonidine was replaced by the transdermal preparation, have shown that antihypertensive efficacy can be maintained despite a marked reduction in plasma clonidine concentrations. From a historical perspective, it is interesting that as we become more familiar with antihypertensive drugs, we tend to use them in lower doses. This applies to a wide range of drugs, including agents such as reserpine, methyldopa, hydralazine, some of the β-blockers, and the thiazide diuretics, all of which now tend to be used in more modest doses than when they were first made available. This also seems to be true for newer drugs such as captopril. I think that the data presented by Dr. Kolloch, together with our experiences with the transdermal clonidine, have helped to emphasize that a decrease in the previously accepted dosage levels of clonidine will probably not reduce its efficacy but might have a beneficial impact on its side-effect profile.

MATHIAS:

Dr. Lowenthal's data from his patients with renal insufficiency showed that systolic blood pressure was reduced to a much greater extent than diastolic pressure when the patients were supine. Could this mean that in these patients cardiac output was contributing to their blood pressure to a large extent? I think it is established that patients on haemodialysis tend to have increased cardiac output owing to their vascular shunts.

104

LOWENTHAL:

I cannot answer your question directly, because we did not perform invasive haemodynamic studies in these patients. But as you know from the earlier work with clonidine, there is often a reduction in cardiac output early in the course of treatment. We believe that cardiac output does not change appreciably during clonidine therapy in patients with renal insufficiency, and I am not certain whether the large changes in systolic blood pressure can be attributed to this.

Catapres Transdermal Therapeutic System (TTS) for Long-Term Treatment of Hypertension

J. C. Boekhorst[1] and R. G. L. van Tol[2]

Introduction

Short-term studies have shown that the clonidine transdermal therapeutic system (Catapres-TTS) is an effective and safe therapy for treatment of mild to moderate hypertension. Frequency and intensity of systemic side-effects appeared to be less than those experienced during conventional oral antihypertensive treatment. Local skin reactions reported during short-term TTS treatment were mainly periods of itching and erythema at the TTS site. Skin reactions usually disappeared within two days of removal of the patch. Several patients developed an allergic skin reaction of the delayed type (type IV). Data on long-term treatment with Catapres-TTS are necessary to establish the value of this new therapeutic approach in essential hypertension. The aim of this study was to evaluate efficacy and safety of Catapres-TTS, during a period of treatment of one year in maintaining control of raised blood pressure in mild to moderate hypertensive patients who have been controlled on oral clonidine (Catapres) and a diuretic.

Patients and Methods

Twenty patients (aged 32–76, average 58.8), five males and 15 females, with mild to moderate hypertension controlled on oral clonidine (maximum 0.45 mg/day) and a diuretic were studied. Exclusion criteria were: evidence of clinically relevant cardiac, haematological, renal, hepatic, metabolic or neoplastic disease, cutaneous disorders of any type; history of skin allergy, pregnant or lactating women, use of major tranquillizers. Oral clonidine was replaced by Catapres-TTS, and patients were titrated with a maximum of three units (3.5 cm²) applied once weekly. Blood pressure, pulse rate, safety and clonidine plasma levels were evaluated at regular intervals during oral clonidine treatment, and during titration, four weeks of stable dose and continued long-term Catapres-TTS therapy. Clonidine plasma concentrations were measured with a specific radioimmunoassay. Catapres-TTS, 3.5 cm² in area, contains ± 2.5 mg clonidine, of which approximately 45% is delivered during seven days of wearing.

---

[1] Department of Internal Medicine, Ikazia Hospital, Rotterdam, and
[2] Clinical Research Department, Boehringer Ingelheim bv, Alkmaar, The Netherlands.

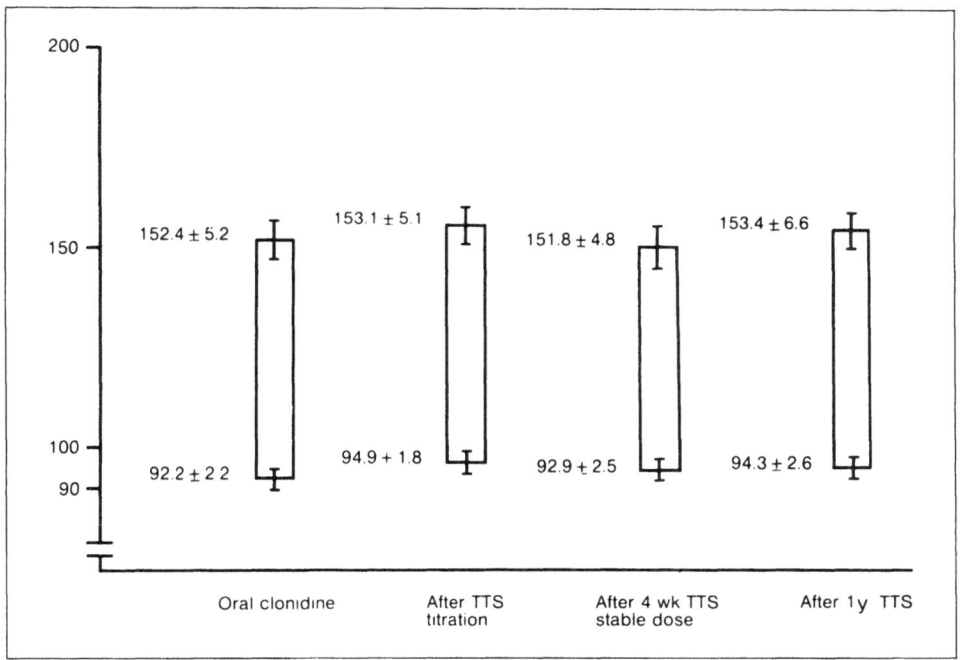

Fig. 1. Sitting Blood Pressure (mmHg) mean values (N = 17) ± SEM.

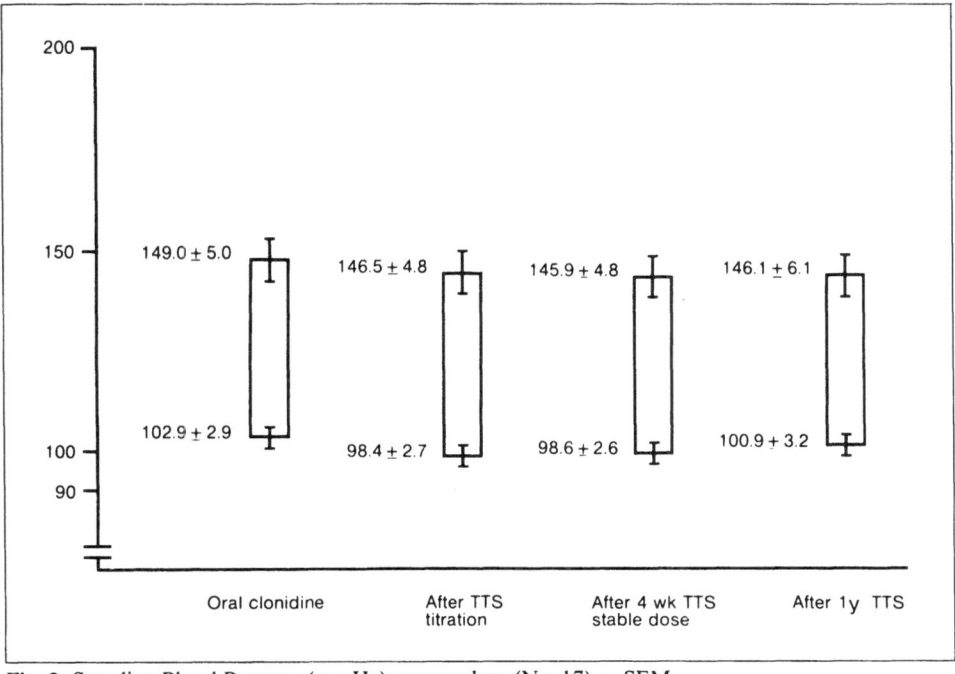

Fig. 2. Standing Blood Pressure (mmHg) mean values (N = 17) ± SEM.

Results

All 20 patients completed titration and four weeks of stable dose TTS treatment and preferred to continue this therapy. Seventeen patients completed one year of TTS treatment and three patients dropped out of the study.

Table 1. Dosage of Catapres-TTS necessary to achieve and maintain blood pressure control (in combination with diuretics and possibly other antihypertensive medication).

	Catapres-TTS (3.5 cm²)	
	No. of patients (N)	No. of units per wk*
During 4 wk TTS stable does treatment (N = 20)	10	1
	5	2
	5	3
After 1 year TTS treatment (N = 17)	5	1
	4	2
	8	3
Changes in dosage of TTS	1	1 → 2 units
	2	1 → 3 units
	1	2 → 3 units

* During long-term treatment also systems of 7.0 and 10.5 cm² have been used. In this table, systems of 7.0 and 10.5 cm² are considered as 2, respectively 3 units.

Table 2. Clonidine plasma concentrations during oral and transdermal Catapres treatment. (Of nine patients with unchanged antihypertensive medication during long-term TTS stable dose treatment.)

Patient no.	Oral Clonidine		Catapres-TTS Plasma (ng/ml)			
	Dose (mg)	Plasma (mg/ml)	(nits TTS)	Titration	4 wks	1 Year
1	0.300	2.515	1	0.490	0.470	0.285
2	0.150	0.335	1	0.305	0.325	0.235
6	0.450	0.965	1	0.245	0.280	0.600
7	0.150	0.795	1	0.545	0.380	0.110
11	0.450	0.335	2	0.310	0.320	0.310
12	0.300	2.220	2	0.335	0.705	1.490
18	0.150	0.940	3	1.995	2.225	0.600
19	0.450	2.075	3	–	1.820	1.545
20	0.450	2.245	3	–	1.640	1.700
×(N = 9)	0.317	1.381	1.9	–	0.907	0.764
± SEM	0.046	0.291	0.3	–	0.255	0.211

Efficacy

There was no significant difference between controlled blood pressure values during oral clonidine, when compared to blood pressure values during TTS treatment (titration, four weeks of stable dose and one year). To maintain adequate blood pressure control during long-term TTS, the following changes in antihypertensive medication were made: increase of TTS dosage in two patients (Table 1); increase of TTS dosage plus additional antihypertensive medication in two patients (Table 1); additional antihypertensive medication in three patients. In 10 patients there was no change in antihypertensive medication during the one year study period.

Clonidine plasma concentration

Mean steady state clonidine plasma concentrations in a group of nine patients with unchanged antihypertensive medication after four weeks and one year of TTS treatment were respectively 0.907 ng/ml and 0.764 ng/ml. Mean steady state clonidine plasma concentration during oral clonidine in this group was 1.381 ng/ml.

Side-effects

Eleven patients on oral Catapres and 2 patients on Catapres-TTS reported systemic side-effects (Table 3). Local side-effects are shown in Table 4.

Drop-outs

Three patients dropped out of the studyf after a maximum of seven months on Catapres-TTS (Table 5).

Table 3. Systemic side-effects reported during stable dose oral Catapres and stable dose Catapres-TTS.

Oral Catapres	Catapres-TTS
N = 8, Dry mouth moderate-severe	N = 1, Dry mouth
N = 3, Sedation mild-moderate	N = 1, Nervous
N = 3, Headache mild-severe	
N = 2, Bitter-dirty taste severe	
N = 1, Dizziness severe	

Table 4. Local side-effects during treatment with Catapres-TTS*.

Catapres-TTS Titration	Catapres-TTS Stable Doses
N = 4, Erythema definite	N = 2, Erythema Mild-definite
N = 3, Itching mild	N = 1, Itching severe
	N = 3, Contact allergy 2 patients dropped out 1 patient continued

* Mainly all reactions observed and reported were at the site of application of Catapres-TTS.

Table 5. Drop-outs during one year of treatment with Catapres-TTS.

Patient no.	Months of treatment with TTS	Reason for drop-out
5	4.25	Local skin reaction contact allergy*
9	6	Sick-sinus syndrome
13	7	Local – generalized (arm, abdomen) skin reaction, contact allergy*

* Confirmed by patch-testing

Conclusions

Long-term, at least up to one year, control of raised blood pressure in patients with mild to moderate hypertension achieved with oral clonidine up to 0.45 mg per day, and a diuretic, can also be realised when oral Catapres is replaced by the Catapres-TTS. During one year of Catapres-TTS treatment, steady state therapeutic clonidine plasma levels are maintained, and systemic tolerance is very good. Three of 20 patients had to discontinue TTS therapy, two patients because of contact allergy and one because of sick-sinus syndrome. Contact allergy, confirmed by patch testing, developed during TTS treatment in three of 20 patients (15%). After sensitization one patient continued antihypertensive therapy with TTS, and one patient with oral Catapres, without (clinical) problems. In the other patients local skin tolerance of Catapres-TTS was good. All 17 patients who completed one year of treatment with Catapres-TTS, preferred to continue this therapy.

Authors' address:
J. C. Boekhorst, M.D.
Department of Internal Medicine
Ikazia Hospital
3083 AN Rotterdam
The Netherlands

Transdermal Clonidine/Atenolol in the Management of Mild to Moderate Hypertension

Lindsey Dow and M. Searle

Introduction

The clonidine transdermal therapeutic system (Catapres-TTS) delivers clonidine by diffusion through an adhesive plaster on the skin. It is available in sizes 2.5, 5 and 7 mg to deliver daily 0.1, 0.2, or 0.3 mg clonidine respectively. Steady-state levels are reached in three days. The plaster is changed weekly. There is no withdrawal syndrome as clonidine

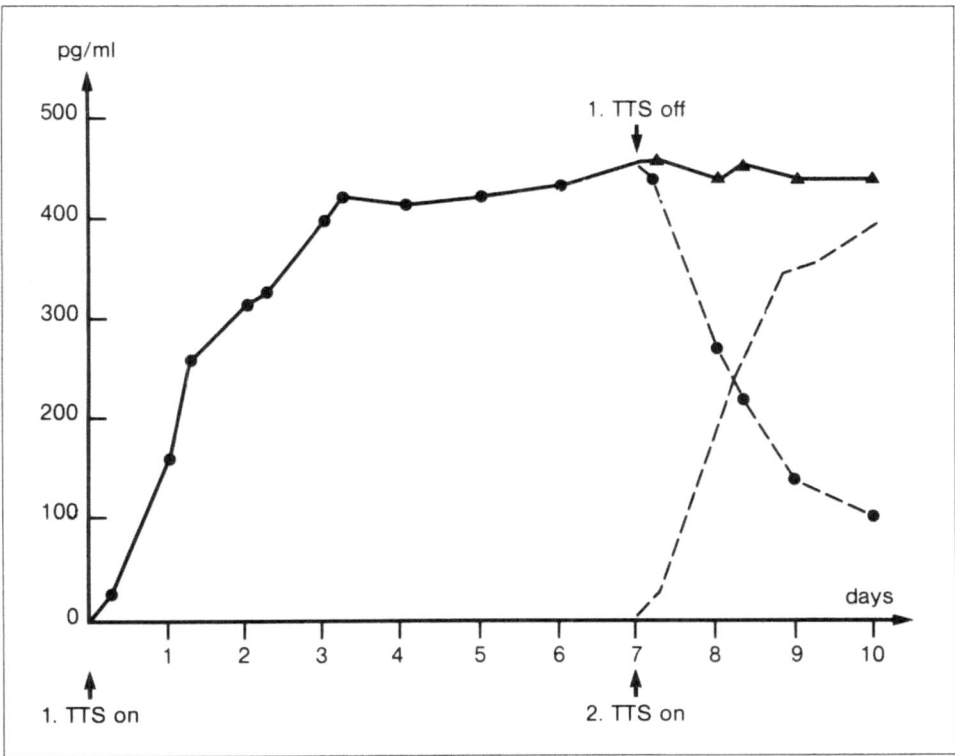

Fig. 1. Simulated plasma clonidine profile following two consecutive applications of clonidine-TTS (5 cm²) on fresh skin sites of the upper outer arm. * Simulated experimental 5 cm²-TTS used on upper outer arm, N = 17. Reproduced by permission of ALZA Corporation, Palo Alto, California, USA (adapted from Fig. 3 in (1)).

Royal South Hants Hospital and Lymington Hospital, Hampshire, U.K.

levels fall slowly after removal of the plaster (Fig. 1) (1). We compared the efficacy of clonidine-TTS with the well-established drugs atenolol and atenolol + chlorthalidone in mild to moderate hypertension.

Patients and Methods

A double-blind trial with randomized control was set up in three centres (Southampton, Lymington and Cardiff) with 60 patients who have mild to moderate hypertension. Mild to moderate hypertension was taken as diastolic blood pressure (DBP) pre-entry being within the range 90–115 mmHg on zero sphygmomanometer on at least two occasions. Exclusion criteria included the following: cardiac, renal, hepatic, metabolic, obstructive airway, neoplastic, haematological and allergic diseases. Patients were referred newly diagnosed from general practitioners or hospital inpatient departments where they had been previously treated; all medication had been stopped two weeks before entry into the trial. The drugs used were clonidine-TTS (2.5/5 mg), atenolol (100 mg), atenolol + chlorthalidone (25 mg). The trial was carried out according to the design in Figure 2.

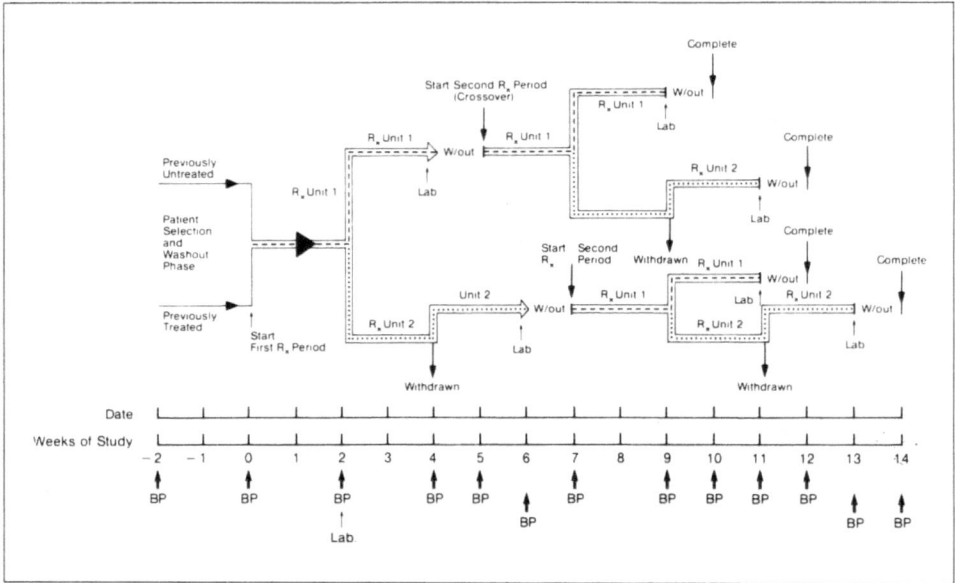

Fig. 2. Clonidine TTS
-------- Unit 1 = Catapres-TTS 1 (Active or placebo)
    +   (Active or placebo)
.... Unit 2 = Catapres-TTS 2 (Active or placebo)
    +   (Active or placebo)

Results

The results from 19 patients to-date are as follows: 12 have completed the trial and seven were withdrawn. The 12 patients had a mean pre-entry BP 174/103 mmHg.

Atenolol/atenolol + chlorthalidone

For four weeks BP was ≤ 140/90 mmHg in six patients (DBP was ≤ 90 mmHg in ten, of whom four had systolic BP (SBP) ≥ 140 mmHg).

Clonidine-TTS 2.5 mg

For four weeks BP was 140/90 mmHg in three patients. (DBP ≤ 90 in four, but SBP was ≥ 140 in one of these four).

Side-effects

Of the 12 patients, 10 reported none on clonidine-TTS and nine none on atenolol/atenolol + chlorthalidone. Side-effects reported from clonidine-TTS were: dry mouth (1), cold numb hands (1), itching at plaster site (1), tiredness (1), irritability (1). Side-effects reported during atenolol/atenolol + chlorthalidone were cold numb hands (2) and impotence (1).

Of the different drugs, 10 patients expressed no preference, one preferred clonidine and one preferred atenolol/atenolol + chlorthalidone. Of the seven patients who were withdrawn from the trial, five had moderate to severe side-effects and in two blood pressure was not controlled. The side-effects were: tiredness/drowsiness (three on clonidine-TTS), depression/irritability (one on clonidine-TTS), dry mouth (one on clonidine-TTS) and tiredness/irritability (one on atenolol/atenolol + chlorthalidone).

Reference

1. Shaw JE, Enscore D, Chu L (1984) Clonidine rate-controlled system: technology and Rinetics. In: Weber MA, Mathias CJ (eds) Mild Hypertension. Steinkopff Verlag Darmstadt, p 134

Authors' address:
Lindsey Dow, M.R.C.P.
Basing Dene Cottage
Privett
Nr. Alton
Hampshire
U.K.

Structure and Function of Catapres-TTS

D. J. Enscore, L. C. Chu, and J. E. Shaw

Introduction

Clonidine is an effective antihypertensive agent which can be taken orally (Shaw et al. 1984). A transdermal therapeutic system (Catapres-TTS) has been developed which when applied to intact skin delivers clonidine to the systemic circulation in a rate-controlled manner for seven days (Shaw et al. 1983). Advantages of Clonidine-TTS include reduction of the daily dosage of drug required to control hypertension, reduction of the frequency and intensity of side-effects, and improved patient compliance in treatment. The transdermal system minimizes the variability in systemic input of drug which could result from the variability in skin permeability, by placing a high percentage of control over the rate of drug delivered to the blood stream, in the dosage form itself.

Dosage form design

Catapres-TTS is a very thin (0.02 cm) flexible film composed of four laminated layers. Proceeding from the visible surface towards the surface attached to the skin, these layers are: 1) a backing layer that provides a physical barrier to loss of drug; 2) a drug reservoir that provides for a continuous supply of drug for one week; 3) a microporous membrane that controls the rate of delivery of clonidine from the drug reservoir to the skin surface and 4) an adhesive formulation containing clonidine that permits passage of the drug from the reservoir and provides effective attachment of the dosage form to the skin. Before use, a release liner, protecting the adhesive, is removed and discarded (Fig. 1).

Fig. 1. Dosage form design of Catapres-TTS.

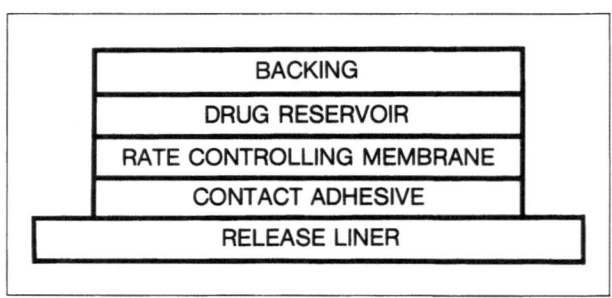

BACKING

DRUG RESERVOIR

RATE CONTROLLING MEMBRANE

CONTACT ADHESIVE

RELEASE LINER

ALZA Corporation, Palo Alto, California, U.S.A.

The chemical potential (concentration) gradient of clonidine effects transfer of drug from the drug reservoir to the surface of the skin. A steady state of clonidine release is derived from the continued maintenance of a saturated solution of clonidine, and the resulting constant thermodynamic potential, within the drug reservoir throughout the one-week lifetime of the system.

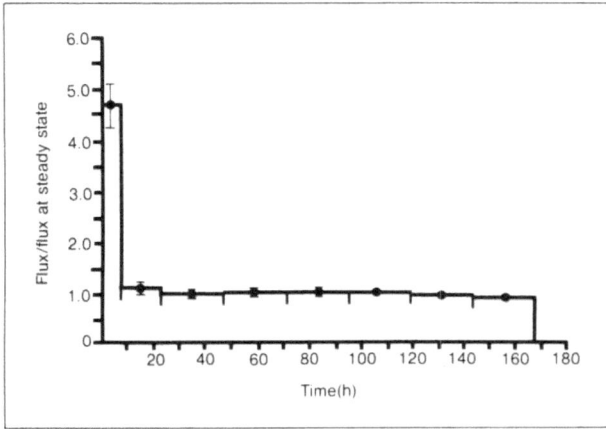

Fig. 2. Rate of release of clonidine from Catapres-TTS at 32 °C into an acidified water receptor solution.

Drug release rates

Initially there is a rapid release of drug from the contact adhesive layer. As the content of the contact adhesive falls below saturation, clonidine is released from the reservoir at a rate predetermined by the properties of the rate-controlling membrane. Thus, from 24 hours through the remainder of the lifetime of the dosage form (168 h), clonidine is released at a constant rate.

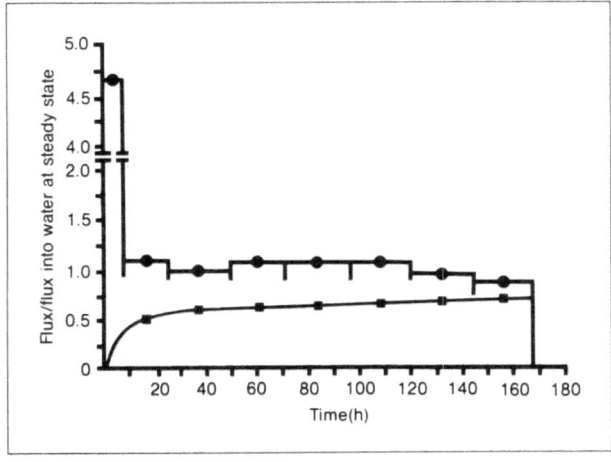

Fig. 3. Rate of clonidine release and rate of permeation of drug through human epidermis.

115

After an initial lag time (reflecting the time during which drug released from the contact adhesive layer is being absorbed into the skin) drug permeation through the skin in vitro reaches a steady rate which is approximately 75% of that released into an infinite sink of water. These data indicate that in vitro the dosage form provides 75% control over the rate of drug permeation through the skin. We have assessed the performance of Catapres-TTS over seven days.

Patients and Methods

During a single seven-day wearing of 5 cm² Catapres-TTS in 17 normal volunteers on the upper outer arm, drug plasma levels rose over 48 h to a steady value which was maintained throughout the seven days of wearing (Fig. 4). Following removal of the dosage form, the plasma levels declined over the next 48 hours. If, at the time the first system was removed, a second system was placed on a fresh skin site, the constancy of drug plasma levels was maintained. The plasma levels associated with wearing of the Catapres-TTS were compared, in the same volunteers, with those resulting from oral administration of 0.1 mg Catapres twice daily (Fig. 5). With both transdermal and oral therapy, there was a reduction in blood pressure. Due to reduction of the daily peaks in plasma drug concentration, a lower incidence and severity of drowsiness and dry mouth were noted during transdermal therapy relative to oral therapy.

The average clonidine plasma concentration measured at steady state (48–168 h) during wearing of different dosages (increasing sizes) of the Catapres-TTS, increase in proportion to the area of skin covered; the plasma levels were directly proportional to the area of the dosage form applied (Shaw 1984).

Conclusions

The Catapres-TTS dosage form provides systemic input of clonidine at a predetermined, constant rate for one week. The rate-controlling membrane in the Catapres-TTS controls

Fig. 4. Plasma clonidine levels in 17 subjects wearing a single 5 cm² Catapres-TTS over seven days.

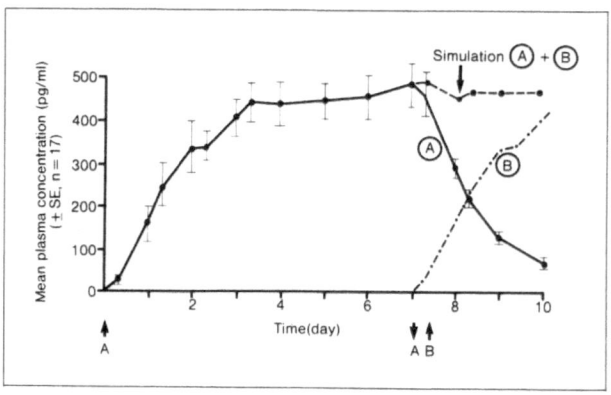

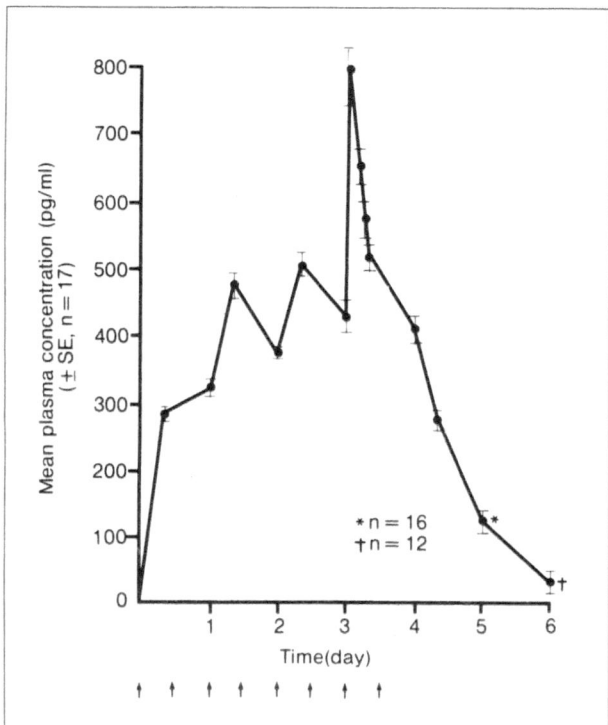

Fig. 5. Plasma clonidine levels in the same 17 subjects given 0.1 mg oral Catapres twice daily over six days.

the rate of drug input to the blood stream, minimizing the intra- and inter-patient variability in the dose of drug received which could result if skin, with its inherent variability in permeability, were allowed to control the rate of drug input. The rate of drug input from Catapres-TTS is directly proportional to the area of the dosage form applied to the skin.

References

1. Shaw JE, Gale RM, Enscore DJ, Chu LC (1983) Predictable percutaneous absorption presented at 10th International Symposium on Controlled Release of Bioactive Materials, San Francisco, USA
2. Shaw JE (1984) Pharmacokinetics of nitroglycerin and clonidine delivered by the transdermal route. Am Heart J 109: 217–223
3. Shaw JE, Enscore D, Chu L (1984) Clonidine rate-controlled system: technology and kinetics. In: Weber MA, Mathias CJ (eds) Mild Hypertension. Steinkopff, Darmstadt p 134–142

Authors' address:
D. J. Enscore, Ph.D.
ALZA Corporation
Palo Alto, California
U.S.A.

117

Interaction of Clonidine and Beta Blocking Agents in the Treatment of Essential Hypertension

R. Fogari and L. Corradi

Introduction

The co-administration of clonidine and β-blockers is usually avoided because it might produce a deleterious interaction resulting in the loss of hypertensive control. However, evidence of this harmful interaction is based largely on one report by Saarimaa (1976). Few other studies have been made, particularly on whether this association is deleterious with all β-blockers or only with some of them. Recent reports suggest that the cardioselective β-blockers do not interact negatively with clonidine. We compared the blood pressure response to the co-administration of clonidine and cardioselective and non-cardioselective β-blockers in essential hypertension.

Patients and Methods

The study was carried out in 25 essential hypertensives (WHO I-II, aged 39–61 years) who were selected from 32 outpatients previously randomised to one of the three different antihypertensive treatments according to the trial design (Fig. 1). Twenty-five subjects failed to reach a diastolic blood pressure below 95 mmHg with any of the three drugs (clonidine 0.075 mg twice a day, atenolol 50 mg once a day, nadolol 40 mg once a day). They were treated with clonidine in combination with both nadolol and atenolol at different times, in the same doses, for four weeks. Lying and standing blood pressure and heart rate were monitored the last day of each treatment period.

Results

Combined administration of clonidine and nadolol reduced blood pressure to a level similar to that recorded after either drug alone, by contrast, the combination of clonidine and atenolol caused a significantly greater reduction in both systolic and diastolic blood pressure compared to the pressures recorded at the end of treatment with either clonidine alone ($p < 0.01$) or atenolol alone ($p < 0.05$). (Table 1, Figs. 1 and 2). Further, with combined administration of clonidine and atenolol a higher percentage of patients

Department of Internal Medicine and Therapeutics, University of Pavia, Pavia, Italy

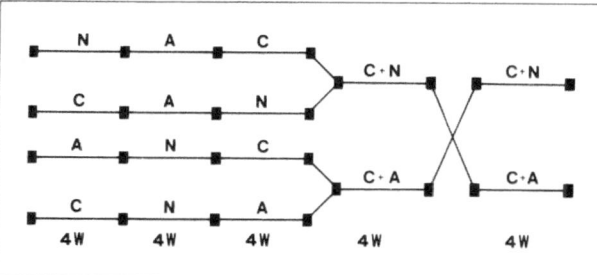

Fig. 1. Design of the trial. C = clonidine, A = atenolol, N = nadolol.

Table 1. Haemodynamic effects of the different treatments (Mean ± SD).

Treatment	Supine			Standing		
	SBP	DBP	HR	SBP	DBP	HR
Control	190 ± 25	118 ± 15	81 ± 9	179 ± 23	124 ± 16	92 ± 10
Clonidine	164 ± 19	104 ± 13	70 ± 10	156 ± 20	106 ± 11	78 ± 8
Nadolol	160 ± 18	104 ± 10	64 ± 8	155 ± 17	110 ± 10	66 ± 6
Atenolol	155 ± 17	101 ± 11	62 ± 7	149 ± 17	105 ± 11	63 ± 7
Clonidine + nadolol	162 ± 19	105 ± 13	57 ± 8	157 ± 18	111 ± 12	62 ± 8
Clonidine + atenolol	143 ± 20	94 ± 10	58 ± 8	138 ± 16	99 ± 9	61 ± 7

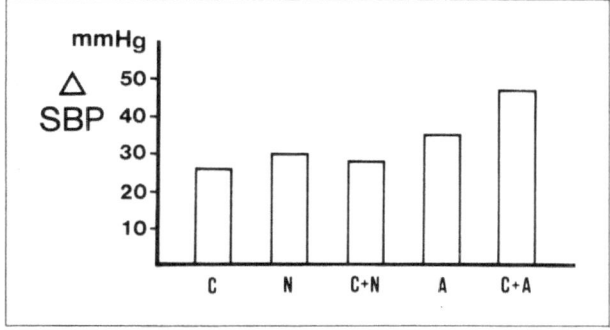

Fig. 2. Systolic blood pressure decrease with the different treatments. C = clonidine, A = atenolol, N = nadolol.

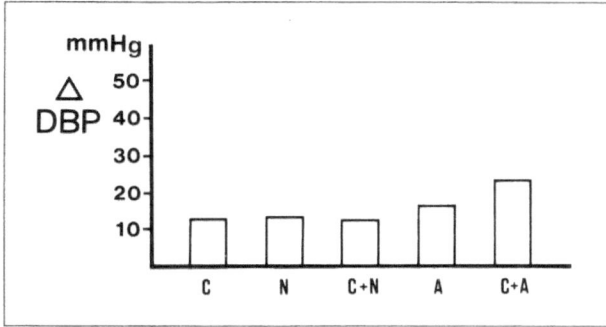

Fig. 3. Diastolic blood pressure decrease with the different treatments. C = clonidine, A = atenolol, N = nadolol.

119

reached a supine diastolic blood pressure below 95 mmHg (Fig. 4). The bradycardic effect of clonidine was enhanced in the same way by the concomitant administration of the two β-blockers; in both cases, however, no patient developed such a slow heart rate as to warrant stopping the treatment. No new side-effect was observed during treatment periods when β-blockers were added to clonidine.

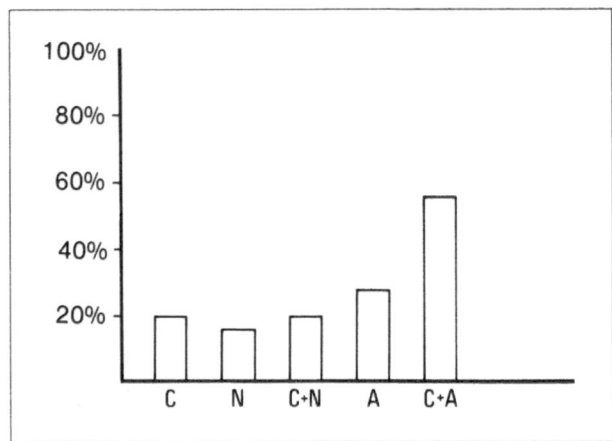

Fig. 4. Percentage of hypertensive who reached a diastolic of blood pressure < 95 mmHg. C = clonidine, A = atenolol, N = nadolol.

Conclusions

These results show that in essential hypertension concomitant administration of atenolol and clonidine significantly decreases both systolic and diastolic blood pressures more than when the two drugs are given separately. By contrast the administration of clonidine and nadolol shows no additive effect; however, there is no loss of pressure control. The following conclusions may be drawn: the lack of additive action between clonidine and non-selective nadolol suggests that peripheral β_2-receptors are involved: the non-selective β-blockers, when opposing the β_2-mediated vasodilation, could constrict blood vessels. This fact, as well as the possible peripheral action of clonidine, may increase the total peripheral resistance which counteracts the additive hypotensive action of the two drugs. The finding that concomitant administration of clonidine and nadolol does not produce a rise in blood pressure is not in agreement with the clinical findings of Saarimaa, but it does agree with Lilja's report (1980) where propranolol was used. This suggests that Saarimaa's results may be attributed to a non-specific property of sotalol. The finding that the combined application of clonidine and atenolol, at least in low doses, enhances the antihypertensive effect of the single drugs is very important particularly because it provides a further treatment combination in the therapy of hypertension and it allows a smaller dose of clonidine, therefore decreasing its troublesome side-effects such as sedation and dry mouth. Furthermore this combination seems to be safe and devoid of dangerous side-effects.

120

References

1. Lilja M, Jounela AJ, Juustila H, Mattila MJ (1980) Interaction of clonidine and β-blockers. Acta Med Scand 207: 173–176
2. Saarimaa H (1976) Combination of clonidine and sotalol in hypertension. Br Med J 1: 810

Authors' address:
R. Fogari, M.D.
Department of Internal Medicine
and Therapeutics
University of Pavia
Pavia
Italy

Catapres-TTS Monotherapy for the Treatment of Mild Hypertension in General Practice: A Preliminary Report

G. S. M. Kellaway and W. F. Lubbe

To evaluate the efficacy, side-effects and patient acceptability, compliance and tolerance to Catapres-TTS as monotherapy for the treatment of mild hypertension in general practice.

Patients and Methods

Trial design

Single blind during placebo period; then open label.
Medication: Catapres-TTS-1 containing 2.5 mg clonidine.

Patients

Patients under 70 years of age with mean seated diastolic blood pressure (SDBP) between 90–104 mmHg on three separate visits. Exclusion criteria included evidence of cardiac, renal, hepatic, metabolic or neoplastic disease; skin diseases of any type; history or presence of any skin allergies; pregnancy. Aim 100 subjects.

Method

Placebo TTS for two weeks was followed by a titration period with dosage adjustment as necessary, from one to three patches. "Non responders" with three patches were withdrawn from the study. Blood pressure (BP) control was defined as reduction in SDBP below 90 mmHg. Effective dosage was maintained for a minimum of three months, longer if desired by patients or investigators.
Physical examination and laboratory tests, including haematology, blood chemistry and urinalysis, were undertaken at beginning and end of the study. At each visit BP and pulse were recorded in sitting and standing positions. Patients were questioned about systemic side-effects and observations were made for local skin reactions. Analysis was undertaken with paired t-test.

Auckland, New Zealand.

Fifty-three patients entered and 37 completed the study. Their distribution, response and number of patches are summarised in Table 1. Blood pressure control was achieved in 32 of 36 patients (89%) who completed the titration phase (Fig. 1). Values at the end of titration, one month, two months, and three months were significantly reduced ($p < 0.0005$), from placebo baseline. There were no significant BP level differences between values at one, two, and three months compared to end of titration. At six months (N = 7) sitting and standing diastolic blood pressures were statistically significantly reduced compared with placebo baseline. Sixteen, eight and eight patients required one, two and three Catapres-TTS-1 respectively. At three months 26 patients remained controlled and contin-

Table 1. Patient distribution (N = 37).

Patients dropped during titration		Patients controlled on	
Side-effects	1	1 system	16
Non-responders	4	2 systems	8
Controlled at end of titration	32	3 systems	8

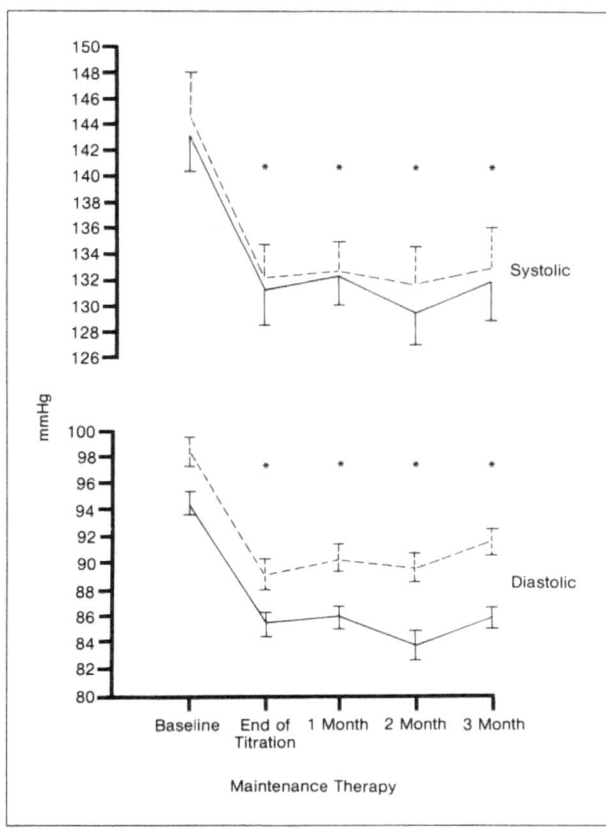

Fig. 1. Mean sitting and standing blood pressure (mmHg) over time for all patients controlled on Catapres-TTS. * p <0.0005). O----O standing. O———O sitting.

123

Table 2. Local adverse effects (N = 37).

Classification of local adverse effects			Severity		
			Mild	Moderate	Severe
Itching:	Baseline	5	5	–	–
	Treatment	15	6	5	4
			Barely perceptible redness	Definite redness	Bright redness
Erythema:	Baseline	10	9	1	–
	Treatment	18	2	8	8
Oedema:	Baseline	–			
	Treatment	12			

Table 3. Patient withdrawals.

Before completion of 3 months' treatment (N = 53)		After 3 months' treatment (N = 26)	
Withdrawals	11	Stopped Catapres-TTS	7
Reasons:			
Allergic skin reaction	5	Allergic skin reaction	7
Non-responders	4	Systemic side-effects	1
Systemic side-effects	1	No specific reason	1
No specific reason	1		

Table 4. Patient assessment.

	Replies N = 45 (92%)					
	Patients without skin reaction			Patients reporting skin reaction		
	Yes	No	Don't Know	Yes	No	Don't Know
Do you find TTS patches easy to use?	25	–	–	20	–	-
Do you prefer once weekly TTS application to more frequent oral (daily or twice daily) pills to control your blood pressure?	24	1	–	15	1	4
Do you understand how your TTS patch works in controlling your blood pressure?	24	–	1	16	2	2
Does TTS irritate your skin?	–	25	–	18	2	–
Do you wish to continue treatment with TTS?	22	2	1	10	8	2

ued into the next three months. There was a minor but significant reduction in heart rate of four to six beats per minute on treatment.

Comparison of systemic side-effects during placebo wash-out period and treatment showed dry mouth and possibly lethargy as dose dependent drug effects. Table 2 summarises local skin reactions which led to withdrawal of five patients from therapy up to three months and a further five patients after three months of treatment (Table 3). In seven of these 10 patients reactions have been confirmed as contact allergies to clonidine. Five were challenged with oral clonidine with no recurrence of skin reaction. Table 4 sumarises patient experience with the use of Catapres-TTS in mild hypertension.

Conclusion

Catapres-TTS has proved effective in controlling mild hypertension with excellent patient acceptability. A tendency for it to produce skin reactions requires further definition to determine exact incidence.

Authors' address:
G. S. M. Kellaway, M.D.
Auckland
New Zealand

Clonidine and Placental Perfusion

N. Pateisky

Introduction

Opinions vary on the use of drugs like clonidine, which may reduce cardiac output and therefore placental perfusion during treatment of pregnancy-induced hypertension; we therefore carried out this retrospective study to determine the influence of clonidine on utero-placental blood flow, by placental perfusion measurement using indium-113 m labelled transferrin, introduced and evaluated in our Department (Leodolter and Philipp 1983).

Patients and Methods

Forty patients (aged 18–43 years) with moderate hypertension, including oedema, proteinuria and hypertension (28–39th week of gestation), were treated with clonidine. The daily oral dose was between 0.15 mg and 0.30 mg. Placental blood flow was measured to study the effect of clonidine on utero-placental blood flow. For the clinical evaluation of the placental perfusion the time-activity curve over the placenta is recorded by means of a gamma scintillation camera after intravenous application of 0.300 mCi [^{113m}In] transferrin. The flow curves (Fig. 1), which are calculated by iterative regression, give good clinical correlation to three perfusion types: type I, unimpaired flow; type II, transitional type: type III, strongly reduced flow.

Results

Table 1 shows the influence of clonidine therapy on the gestosis index. During treatment 10 patients showed a moderate gestosis with an index of 4–7, while 20 patients showed an index of 4–7 before starting clonidine therapy. The reduction in the gestosis index is statistically significant.

The results of placental perfusion measurement during clonidine treatment in three patients showed a type III (strongly reduced flow) and in 12 patients a type II (transitional type). In 25 women a normal type I was recorded, indicating an unimpaired utero-placental perfusion. In 11 patients the perfusion measurement was performed before as well as during clonidine treatment. Table 2 shows that the pattern of perfusion type distribution during treatment with clonidine differs significantly from that before treatment of hypertension.

1st Department of Gynaecology and Obstetrics, Vienna, Austria.

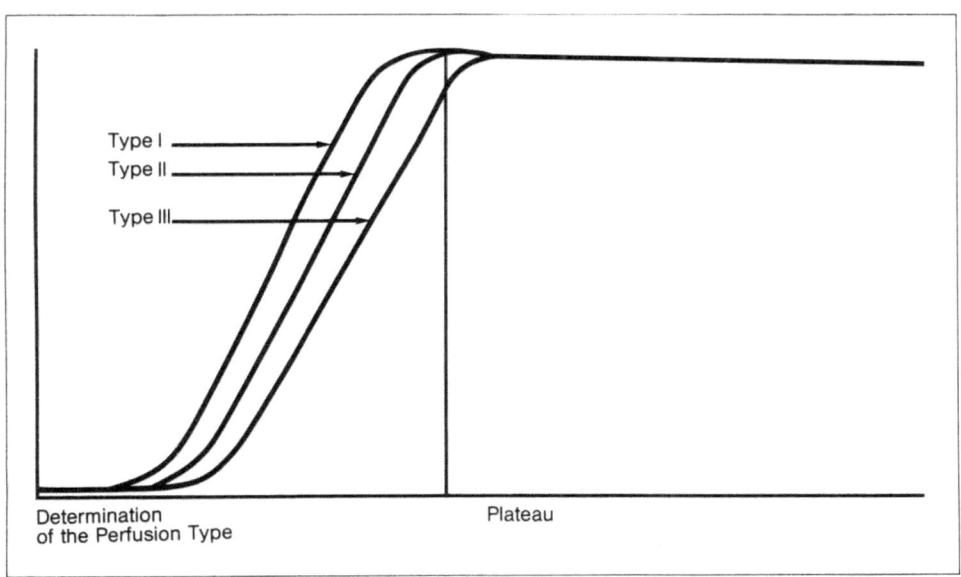

Fig. 1. Time-activity curves of [^{113m}In] transferrin.

Table 1. Gestosis index of 40 patients before and during treatment with clonidine.

	Gestosis Index			
	N	0	1–3	4–7
Before clonidine	40	0	20	20
During clonidine	40		17	10

$X^2 = 16.567$; $p < 0.01$

Table 2. Perfusion type before and during treatment with clonidine.

	Perfusion Type			
	N	I	II	III
Before clonidine	11	3	4	4
During clonidine	40	25	12	3

$x^2 = 7.2981$; $p < 0.05$

The correlation of the perfusion type of the birth-weight of the later born babies was also satisfactory.

127

Conclusions

Since mechanisms of placental perfusion are not yet completely understood, no one can predict exactly the effect of an antihypertensive drug to the utero-placental blood flow. Our data on placental perfusion measurement before and/or during clonidine treatment of pregnant women with moderate EPH-gestosis suggest that oral treatment of pregnancy-induced hypertension with clonidine improves placental perfusion rather than reducing utero-placental blood flow and that clonidine provides a drug of choice for the oral treatment of hypertension in pregnancy in patients with moderate EPH-gestosis.

Reference

1. Leodolter S, Philipp K (1983) Estimation of the uteroplacental perfusion by the use of 113m-In-transferrin and an iterative method. Gynecol and Obstet Invest 16: 172–179

Author's address:
N. Pateisky, M.D.
1st Department of Gynaecology
and Obstetrics
Spitalgasse 23
1090 Vienna
Austria

Effects of Low Oral Clonidine Doses in the Therapy of Mild Hypertension

H. Pozenel

Introduction

The aim of this study was to establish the efficacy of very low doses of clonidine in the therapy of mild hypertension. Estimation of the effectiveness was by:
1. Several daily indirect blood pressure measurements (supine/upright).
2. Directly recorded circadian blood pressure rhythms over 24 hours by radiotelemetry.

Patients and Methods

Twelve male hypertonic patients in WHO stage I/II of their hypertension with diastolic pressure to a maximum of 105 mmHg were studied (Tables 1 and 2). In the pre-treatment period the blood pressure values were about 160/95 mmHg. The pre-treatment period lasted over seven days without any therapy and was continued over 14 days with 0.0375 mg clonidine 12 hourly, followed by a 7-day post-therapy period. On the last day of therapy and the last day of the post-therapy period a 24 h blood pressure telemetry was performed. Several daily blood pressure measurements were taken with an automatic ultrasound apparatus (Arteriosonde) in the morning (6.00 h–7.00 h) before and two hours after the oral doses of clonidine/placebo in the supine and two minutes in the upright standing position (Table 3, Figs. 1 and 2).

Table 1. 12 male hypertonic patients (I/II WHO).

	Range:	Mean ($\pm$ SD)
Age (y):	48–55	51.6 ± 2.4
Height (cm):	153.183	168.3 ± 8.2
Weight (kg):	60–83	72.9 ± 6.7

Herz- und Kreislaufzentrum der Bauern, 4540 Bad Hall, Austria.

Table 2. Diagnosis of patients.

Concomitant diseases:
    1 diabetes mellitus (on diet only)
    4 struma nodosa (without dysfunction)
    2 chronic bronchitis

Additional therapy:
    12 physical therapy
    1 diabetes diet
    1 sulphonamide therapy (chronic bronchitis)

Table 3. Differences in blood pressure (mmHg).

	Supine	Upright
Systolic blood pressure:		
Decrease pre-treatment/therapy period:	9.6 (p = 0.04)	12.9 (p = 0.05)
Increase therapy/post-treatment period:	14.2 (p = 0.02)	21.3 (p = 0.005)
Diastolic blood pressure:		
Decrease pre-treatment/therapy period:	11.2 (p = 0.002)	14.2 (p = 0.003)
Increase therapy/post-treatment period:	10.8 (p = 0.002)	12.1 (p = 0.01)
Decrease 2 h after 0.0375 mg clonidine:	23.7 (p = 0.001)	20.4 (p = 0.004)
Increase 2 h after placebo:	22.5 (p = 0.005)	19.2 (p = 0.02)
Diastolic blood pressure:		
Decrease 2 h after 0.0375 mg clonidine:	14.2 (p = 0.002)	12.9 (p = 0.005)
Increase 2 h after placebo:	14.6 (p = 0.001)	12.9 (p = 0.003)

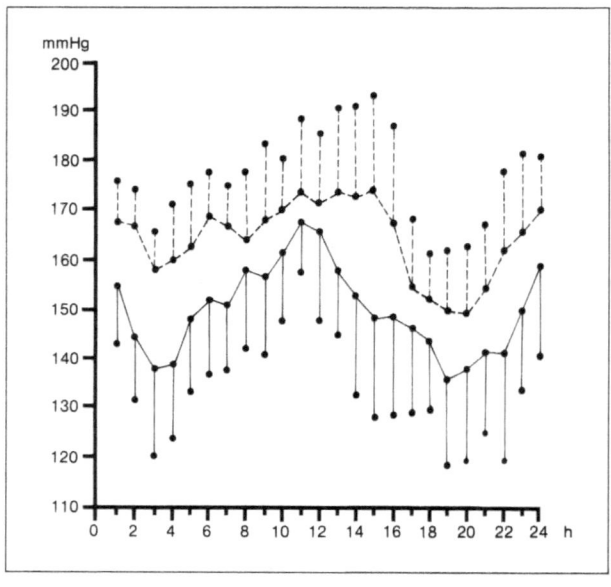

Figs. 1 and 2. Indirect measurements of blood pressure (systolic/diastolic) (mean ± SD) from 12 hypertonics (supine) during study with clonidine (2 × 0.0375 mg) – before and --- after oral dose.

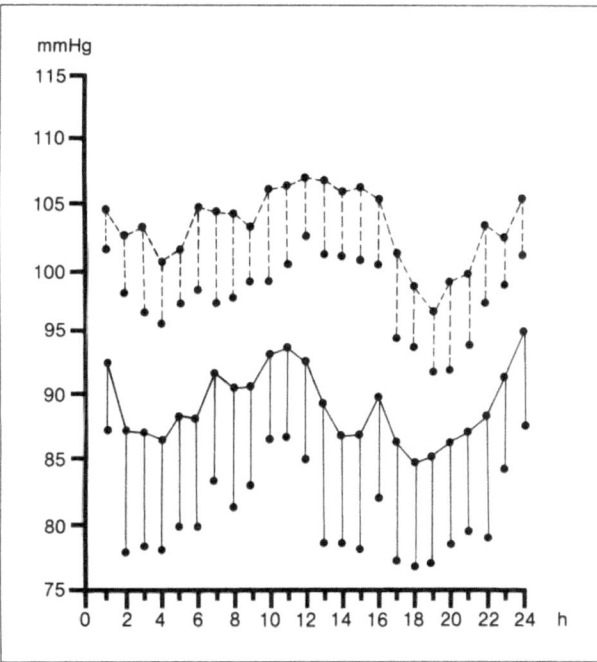

Fig. 2.

Blood pressure profiles were obtained from the brachial artery (Figs. 3 and 4). After insertion of a Teflon catheter (Seldocath n. Grandjean 4F) the blood pressure was amplified by radiotelemetry (Glonner Gemtel TTX 12) and recorded on a Hewlett-Packard 3960

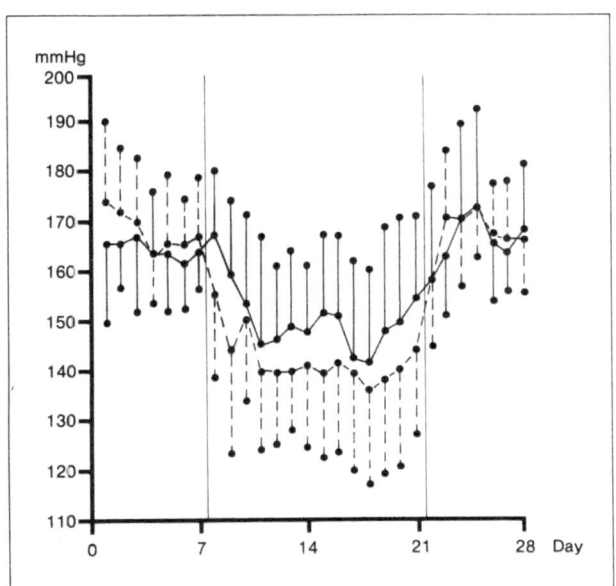

Figs. 3 and 4. Blood pressure profile over 24 h (mean ± SD) of 12 hypertonics. Telemetric values from 7.00 h 7.00 h next day in the post-treatment period (---- and the therapy period with 2 × 0.0375 mg clonidine (–).

Fig. 4.

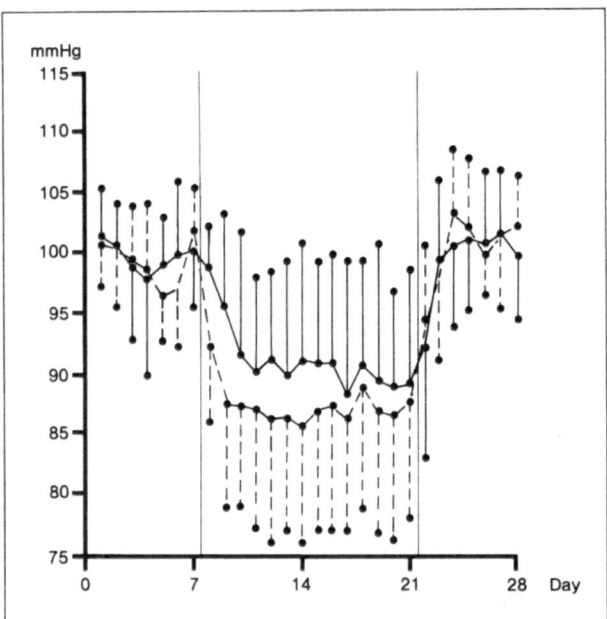

tape-recorder over a period of 24 hours. Compressed blood pressure curves were further analysed at intervals of an hour.

Statistical evaluation of the blood pressure values was performed by comparison of the values at the end of the pre-treatment period with those at the end of the treatment period and those at the end of the post-treatment period, by sequential analysis of statistical data.

Results

Daily indirect blood pressure measurements (Table 3)

The systolic and diastolic blood pressure values during therapy with twice daily 0.0375 mg clonidine were significantly ($p < 0.05$) different from pre-treatment and post-treatment blood pressures.

The efficacy of a single dose of 0.0375 mg clonidine was detectable in that two hours after oral ingestion systolic and diastolic blood pressures in supine and upright positions were significantly different.

24-hour blood pressure profiles (Figs. 3 and 4)

Systolic and diastolic blood pressures on the last therapy day were significantly different ($p < 0.001$) compared with the values at the end of the post-treatment period. The mean increase in systolic pressure was 14.6 mmHg and in diastolic pressure 8.58 mmHg. Heart rate increased in the post-treatment period by about 5.8 b/min (p < 0.005) (mean). The circadian rhythms were not altered during therapy with clonidine, despite the decrease in blood pressure. With the ingestion of a single dose of clonidine there was a distinct decreasing break in the circadian rhythm over 2–4 hours. With low-dose clonidine there was a return to normotensive blood pressure in two of the 12 patients. In five more patients the systolic pressure decreased by at least 20 mmHg. Ten patients showed a reduction in diastolic pressure of at lest 10 mmHg. The overall efficacy of low-dose therapy with clonidine was shown in 11 of the 12 patients by application of following criteria: normotonic blood pressure on treatment, RR < 140/90 mmHg; decrease systolic RR on treatment, RR > 20 mmHg (supine); decrease systolic RR on treatment, RR > 20 mmHg (upright); decrease diastolic RR on treatment: RR > 10 mmHg (supine); decrease diastolic RR on treatment: RR > 10 mmHg (upright).

Conclusion

A controlled study on 12 mild or borderline hypertonic patients showed the efficacy of low-dose therapy with clonidine (0.0375 mg twice a day) on indirectly and directly measured blood pressure. Blood pressure profiles showed that there was a good reduction in blood pressure in 11 patients. The circadian rhythms were lowered toward a normotensive blood pressure level.

Author's address:
H. Pozenel, M.D.
Herz- und Kreislaufzentrum
4540 Bad Hall
Austria

Absorption and Excretion of Clonidine Following Application of Catapres-TTS to Different Skin Sites

K. Hopkins[1], L. Aarons[2], and M. Rowland[2]

A transdermal therapeutic system is most effective when the rate-controlling step lies primarily in the system rather than in the skin. For this condition to prevail the skin must be sufficiently permeable to the drug. The permeability of the skin at different body sites, however, can vary. We have assessed the influence of site of application to the skin of a transdermal clonidine therapeutic system (Catapres-TTS) on the plasma concentration and urinary excretion of clonidine.

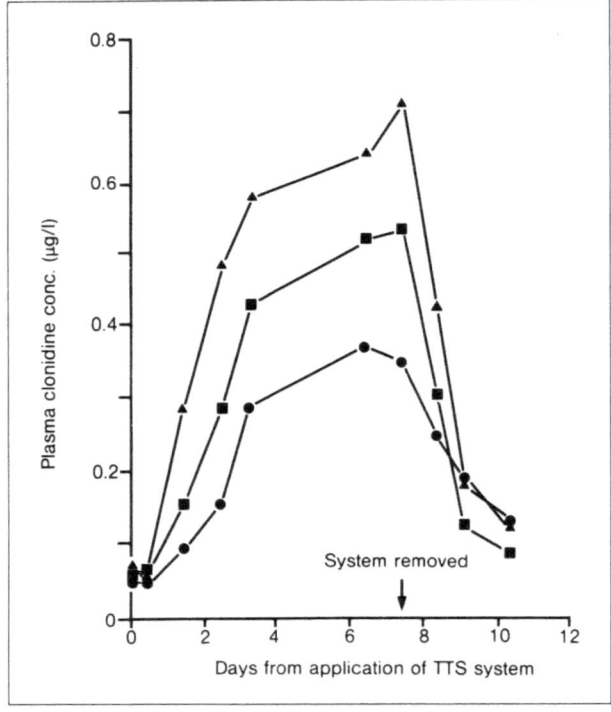

Fig. 1. Mean plasma clonidine concentration during application, and after removal, of Catapres-TTS of different skin sites.

[1] Medical Department, Medeval Limited, University of Manchester and [2] Department of Pharmacy, University of Manchester, Manchester, U.K.

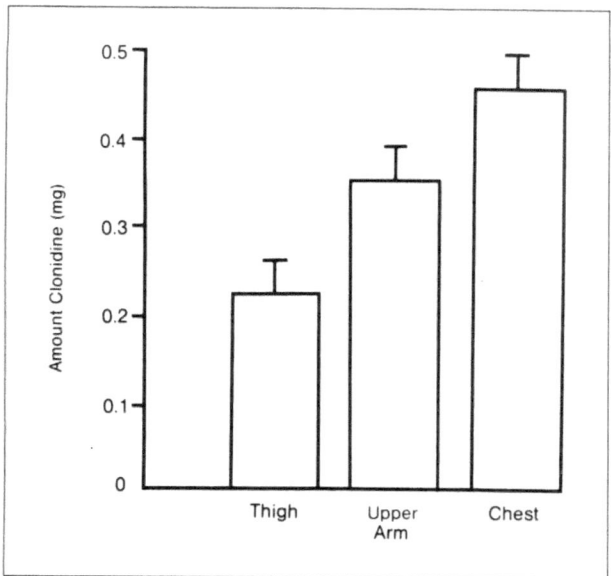

Fig. 2. Mean total (+ SE) urinary excretion of clonidine following application and removal of Catapres-TTS to different skin sites.

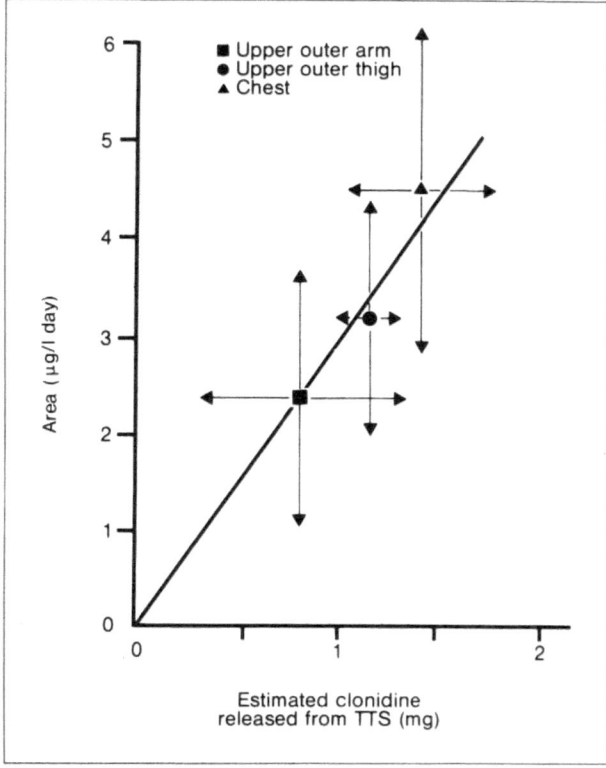

Fig. 3. Correlation between mean amount of clonidine released from the Catapres-TTS and the mean AUC.

Subjects and Methods

Twelve healthy volunteers (nine men, three women, aged 20–39) were studied according to a randomised three-way crossover design. The Catapres-TTS (3.75 cm², designed to release 2.9 µg/h/cm²) was applied to the skin (upper outer arm, upper outer thigh, chest), for one week, with a one-week washout period between applications. Serial blood samples and 24-hour urine collections were taken during and for four days after removal of each transdermal system. Clonidine was analysed in these samples and in the used Catapres-TTS.

Results

The plasma concentration and urinary excretion of clonidine varied with the site of application of the TTS, in the order chest > upper arm > thigh (Figs. 1 and 2). The differences are statistically significant.

A linear correlation was observed between the total area unter the plasma clonidine concentration-time curve (AUC), a measure of bioavailability, and the amount of clonidine released from the Catapres-TTS placed on the different skin sites (Fig. 3). The mean residence time (MRT) of clonidine in the body, in part determined by the absorption time profile of drugs, was significantly longer following application of Catapres-TTS to the upper thigh (mean 5.96 days) than to either the upper arm (mean 5.51 days) or chest (mean

Fig. 4. Correlation between plateau plasma clonidine concentration and AUC.

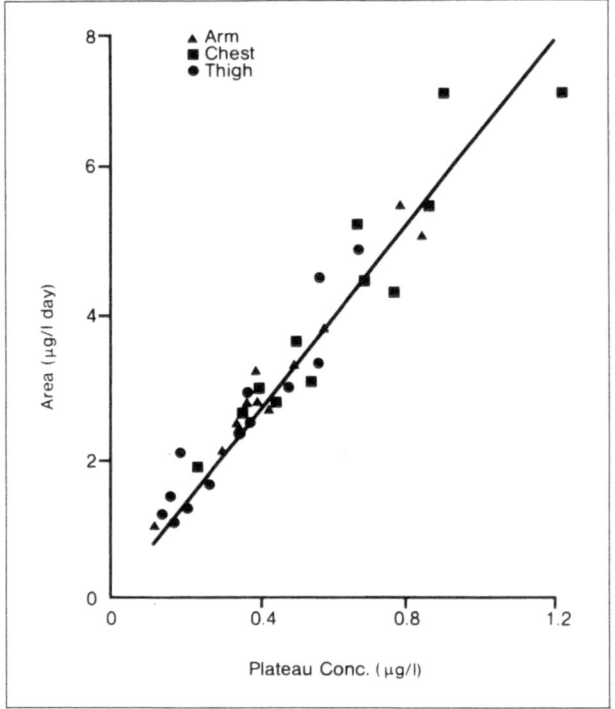

5.36 days). There was linear correlation between the plateau plasma concentration of clonidine (mean of concentration on days 6 and 7) after application and the AUC (Fig. 4).

Conclusions

The permeability of the skin to clonidine varies, with permeability decreasing in the order: chest > upper arm > upper thigh. These differences in skin permeability affect the release of clonidine from the transdermal system. Absorption of clonidine into, and release from the skin of the thigh is slower than from the skin of either the chest or the arm. The plateau plasma clonidine concentration may be a suitable measure of bioavailability when applying Catapres-TTS to the skin.

Authors' address:
K. Hopkins, M.D.
Medical Department
Medeval Limited
Coupland III
University of Manchester
Manchester M13 9PL
U.K.

β-Blockers or Clonidine in Antihypertensive Therapy?

Hermann A. Trauth

Introduction

β-receptor blockers are often considered as agents of first choice in antihypertensive therapy (Kewitz 1978). Side-effects are seldom, contraindications must be noted; in bronchial asthma, β-blockers are contraindicated (Burley 1975; Frishman 1979). We carried out a retrospective investigation of 100 randomly sampled hypertensive patients (bronchial asthma had not been noted in the history) treated with β-blockers and with clonidine. Airway resistance, chest complaints and history of respiratory diseases were compared and the incidence of bronchial side-effects by high-dose (e.g. antihypertensive) β-blocker therapy measured.

Patients and Methods

One hundred randomly sampled patients with hypertension were studied. All had been treated with β-blockers and were referred to us for check-up for various reasons (Tables 2 and 3). We recorded the history of respiratory diseases and complaints, of present complaints and the preliminary interpretation of these complaints. After physical examination a lung function test (whole-body plethysmography) was taken during β-blocker therapy and two to four weeks after changing to clonidine.

Results

We found an unexpectedly high incidence (32%) of increased airway resistance during β-blocker therapy (Table 1). In these cases the subjective complaints together with the primary disease often had suggested a cardiac origin in the preliminary examination (Tables 2 and 3). There was a high incidence of recurrent bronchitis, chronic bronchitis and occurrences of bronchitis in infancy at patients with increased airway resistance (Table 4). There was a significant decrease of airway resistance after change-over to clonidine. Bronchitis and emphysema still had increased airway resistance after the change-over to clonidine, but increase in airway resistance was minimal (Table 5), even if obstructive respiratory disease had not been noted before.

Medizinische Poliklinik Philipps-Universität Marburg, 3550 Marburg, F.R.G.

Table 1. Hypertensive patients treated with β-blockers and clonidine (change-over) – number of cases with increased airway resistance before and after changing over the therapy.

Treated with β-blockers airway resistance increased	N = 32
Treated with clonidine, airway resistance increased	N = 13
Sample of hypertensive patients investigated – total number	N = 100

Table 2. Symptoms – as described by the patients with increased airway resistance.

Hooplike narrowness/feeling of tightness in the chest
Sensitivity of pressure in the chest
Shortness of breathing (of varying intensity or paroxysmal)

Table 3. Preliminary interpretation of the symptoms motive of referral.

Coronary heart disease:	24 ×
myocardial infarction	3 ×
Bronchitis	8 ×
Emphysema	2 ×
"Dyspnoea of unknown origin"	3 ×

Patients with increased airway resistance (N = 32)

Table 4. Bronchitis in infancy and recurrent bronchitis indicates a high risk of bronchial side-effects by antihypertensive therapy with β-blockers.

Previous diseases and signs	Airway resistance (R_t)	
	Increased	Normal
Chronic bronchitis and/ or emphysema	7	6
Allergic rhinitis	1	–
Allergic persons	3	–
Recurrent bronchitis	12	–
Bronchitis in infancy	12	5
Wheezing during bronchitis	28	17

Table 5. The decrease of airway resistance after change-over to clonidine is significant. Increased airway resistance (mean and SD) during β-blocker therapy and after change-over to clonidine.

	Airway resistance (R_t)			
	N	Treated with β-blockers	Treated with clonidine	Decrease
"Cardioselective" β-blockers	5	7.38 + 2.13	4.06 + 1.87	significant (p < 0.05)
Propranolol	27	6.28 + 3.92	3.71+ 1.95	significant (p < 0.01)

Conclusion

Antihypertensive therapy with β-blocking agents tends to induce bronchospasm in subjects with a history of non-obstructive respiratory disease (Waal-Manning 1976; Williams and Millard 1980). Bronchitis in infancy, recurrent bronchitis and chronic bronchitis are indicative of a substantially higher risk of bronchial side-effects by high-dose (e.g. antihypertensive) β-blocker therapy (Table 4). Tightness of the chest with the primary disease often suggested a cardiac origin (Table 3), but our observation suggests that more often they may also be of bronchial origin, caused by therapy when a history of respiratory disease is known. The history of respiratory diseases must be taken exactly before treating with β-blockers. In all cases with a history of chronic or recurrent respiratory disease of bronchitis in infancy, clonidine should be preferred to β-blocking agents in antihypertensive therapy. A further prospective study will investigate airway resistance together with the pulmonary artery and wedge pressure, breathing (type and rhythm) and cardiac rhythm during treatment with β-blockers and clonidine (cross-over study).

References

1. Burley DM (1975) Therapiewoche 25: 4342–346
2. Frishman W et al (1979) Am Heart J 98: 256–262
3. Kewitz H (1978) Medizinische und wirtschaftliche rationale Arzneimitteltherapie. Springer, Berlin
4. Waal-Manning HJ (1976) Drugs 12: 412–441
5. Williams JP, Millard FJC (1980) Thorax 35: 160

Author's address:
Hermann A. Trauth, M.D.
Medizinische Poliklinik der
Philipps-Universität Marburg
3550 Marburg
F.R.G.

Pharmacokinetics of Transdermally Delivered Clonidine

R. G. A. van Wayjen[1], A. van den Ende[1], R. G. L. van Tol[2], T. R. MacGregor[3], J. J. Keirns[3], and K. M. Matzek[3]

Introduction

Catapres Transdermal Therapeutic System (Catepres-TTS) is a tan square unit with rounded corners, composed of a flexible system of membranes which adheres to the skin. Proceeding from the visible surface towards the surface attached to the skin, are four layers: backing layer, drug reservoir of clonidine, rate controlling membrane and contact adhesive with loading dose. Before use, a protective peel strip that covers the contact adhesive is removed. The system provides continuous systemic delivery of clonidine for seven days at an approximately constant rate. Catapres-TTS is indicated in the treatment of mild to moderate hypertension. The aim of this study was to evaluate pharmacokinetic of transdermal clonidine at steady state. Three open label studies were undertaken to assess: (1) dose linearity of increasing sizes of Catapres-TTS; (2) the influence of site (chest and upper outer arm) and duration of application; (3) the influence of system removal and replenishment following three consecutive applications.

Patients and Methods

Dose linearity of the TTS was assessed with application of increasing sizes, 3.5, 7.0 and 10.5 cm², to the upper outer arm of six healthy volunteers (aged 21–31). The influence of site and duration of application on absorption of clonidine was evaluated in eight healthy volunteers (aged 22–28) by application of Catapres-TTS (3.5 cm²) to upper outer arm and chest for 11 days each. The influence of system removal and replenishment was assessed in eight healthy volunteers (aged 22–28) following three consecutive applications (4, 3 and 4 days) of Catapres-TTS (3.5 cm²) to alternate upper outer arms. All volunteers, males, with normal weight and good health as documented by history and physical examination, were hospitalized and resided in a separate clinical pharmacology research unit. Blood samples to determine clonidine plasma concentration were taken. In study (1) in steady state 24 hour urine samples were collected quantitatively. Measurement of clonidine concentration in plasma and urine samples was performed by radioimmunoassay. Pharmacodynamics and safety were monitored closely during all studies.

---

[1] Vereeniging voor Ziekenverpleging, Amsterdam, The Netherlands.
[2] Boehringer Ingelheim bv, Alkmaar, The Netherlands.
[3] Boehringer Ingelheim Ltd. Ridgefield, Connecticut, USA.

Results

Steady state clonidine plasma levels were obtained within 72 hours after application of Catapres-TTS (Fig. 1) and increased linearly with increasing dose (Table 1). Mean steady state plasma concentrations with the 3.5 cm², 7.0 cm² and 10.5 cm² systems were 0.39, 0.84 and 1.12 ng/ml respectively. Clonidine clearance varied widely among individuals (2.6–10.8 l/h, approximately four-fold), but was consistent within each individual. In this study, half-life mean 18.3 h, and clearance of clonidine were independent of the dose of TTS, suggesting linear kinetics of clonidine.

Within 72–96 h after application of TTS to upper outer arm or chest, steady state plasma concentrations of clonidine were achieved. Mean $AUC_{0-168 h}$ and mean clonidine steady state levels (72–168 h) were not significantly different following application of Catapres-TTS (3.5 cm²) to arm or chest (Figs. 2 and 3, Table 2). Mean steady state plasma concentrations (time interval 72–168 h after application) were 0.40 ng/ml for the upper outer arm and 0.39 ng/ml for the chest. There was no significant difference between plasma steady state levels and plasma concentrations at time points 192 and 264 h (four days post labelling). Clonidine plasma concentrations varied widely.

Steady state clonidine plasma levels were achieved within 72 h after application of the first TTS to the upper outer arm (Fig. 4). Mean clonidine plasma concentration at steady state (72–264 h) for all eight subjects was 0.32 ng/ml. Plasma concentration at the time the TTS was removed and clonidine concentration 24 h after application of a new system did not differ significantly in seven of eight subjects.

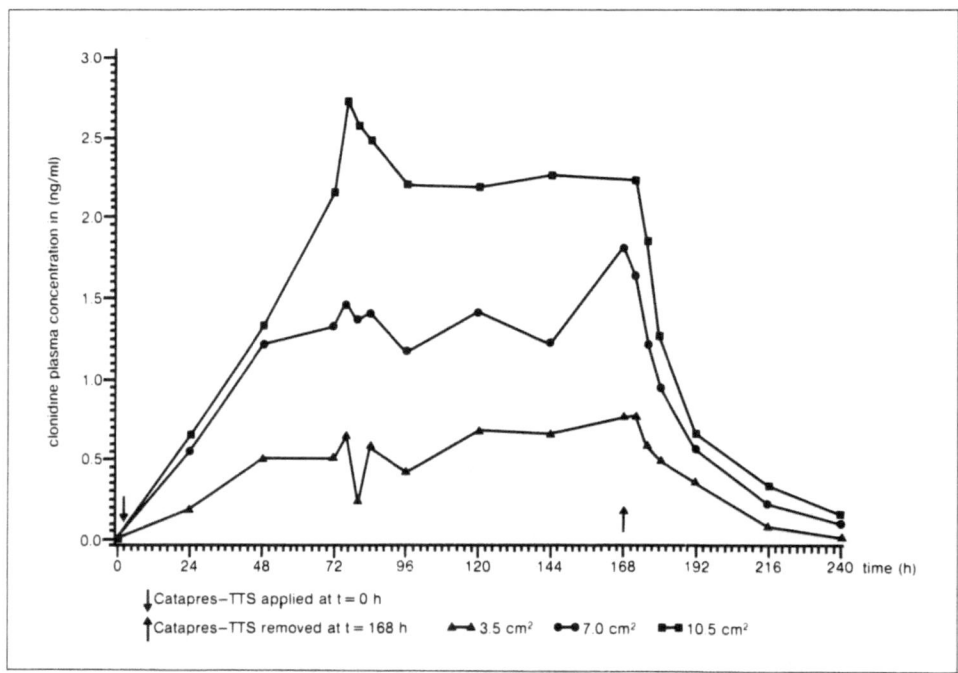

Fig. 1. Time course of clonidine plasma levels in subject 3.

Table 1. Clonidine steady state levels obtained following application of Catapres-TTS 3.5, 7.0 or 10.5 cm² systems.

Subject	Size of system (cm²)	Steady state level (ng/ml)*	Linear correlation of patch size with steady state levels
1	3.5	0.298 ± 0.027	
	7.0	0.791 ± 0.041	0.902
	10.5	0.680 ± 0.056	
2	3.5	0.341 ± 0.068	
	7.0	0.766 ± 0.064	0.999
	10.5	1.145 ± 0.190	
3	3.5	0.631 ± 0.154	
	7.0	1.404 ± 0.301	0.999
	10.5	2.200 ± 0.023	
4	3.5	0.255 ± 0.020	
	7.0	0.461 ± 0.147	0.993
	10.5	0.830 ± 0.268	
5	3.5	0.366 ± 0.028	
	7.0	0.858 ± 0.068	0.975
	10.5	0.965 ± 0.030	
6	3.5	0.431 ± 0.069	
	7.0	0.733 ± 0.128	0.980
	10.5	0.891 ± 0.048	
Mean of 6	3.5	0.387	
	7.0	0.836	
	10.5	1.118	

* Average of plasma concentration days 5, 6, 7 and 8.

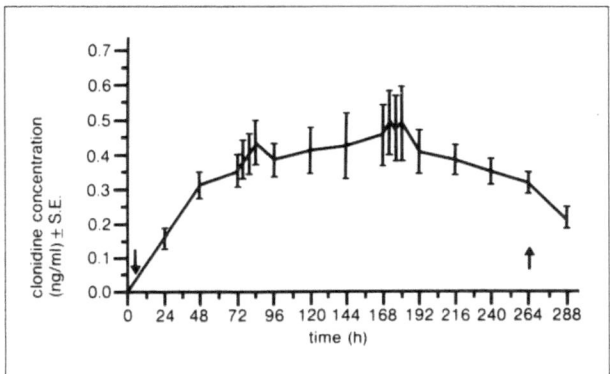

Fig. 2. Mean clonidine plasma concentration following application of Catapres-TTS to the arm; ↓ Catapres-TTS applied at t = 0 h; ↑ Catapres-TTS removed at t = 264 h.

Conclusions

Clonidine was absorbed in a dose-linear manner from TTS in six healthy volunteers. Within each subject the clonidine plasma levels obtained were dose proportional with size of system applied. The high variability among subjects showed that to reach desired

143

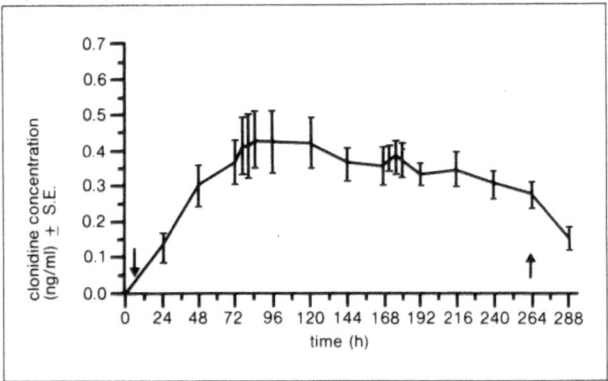

Fig. 3. Mean clonidine plasma concentration following application of Catapres-TTS to the chest; ↓ Catapres-TTS applied at t = 0 h; ↑ Catapres-TTS removed at t = 264 h.

Table 2. Compilation of clonidine steady state plasma concentrations and AUC values obtained following application of TTS-1 (3.5 cm²).

Subject	AUC 0–168 h (ng · h/ml)		Steady state concentration (ng/ml)*	
	Arm	Chest	Arm	Chest
1	24.20	22.54	0.251 ± 0.018	0.232 ± 0.033
2	37.66	41.91	0.366 ± 0.037	0.429 ± 0.046
3	40.59	31.47	0.408 ± 0.032	0.330 ± 0.022
4	27.16	32.48	0.279 ± 0.025	0.333 ± 0.026
5	22.84	16.59	0.238 ± 0.037	0.168 ± 0.026
6	49.09	32.38	0.506 ± 0.069	0.328 ± 0.023
7	78.71	68.78	0.799 ± 0.207	0.707 ± 0.079
8	36.05	58.80	0.377 ± 0.039	0.559 ± 0.191
Mean ± S.D.	38.12 ± 17.7	39.54 ± 18.87	0.403 ± 1.83	0.386 ± 1.75

* Mean 8:00 A.M. plasma clonidine concentration 72–168 h after application of Catapres-TTS-1.

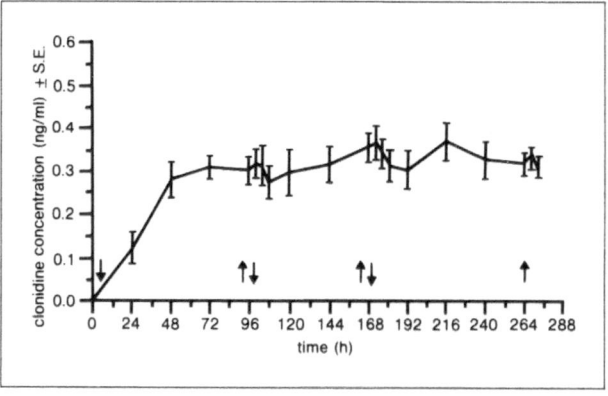

Fig. 4. Mean clonidine plasma concentration following three consecutive applications of Catapres-TTS to the arm; ↓ Catapres-TTS applied at t = 0, 96 and 168 h; ↑ Catapres-TTS removed at t = 96, 168 and 264 h.

144

therapeutic clonidine plasma levels, patients must be titrated with increasing sizes or numbers of Catapres-TTS.

There was no significant influence of site (chest and upper outer arm) or duration of application of Catapres-TTS (3.5 cm^2) on the continued and controlled release of clonidine through the skin for up to 264 h (11 days).

Steady state clonidine plasma levels remain constant upon removal of one system and application of a new system of the same size. Clonidine plasma concentrations at the time a system was removed and a fresh system applied were comparable to plasma concentrations 24 h later.

Authors' address:
R. G. A. van Wayjen, M.D.
Vereeniging voor Ziekenverpleging
Prinsengracht 769
1017 JZ Amsterdam
The Netherlands

Discussion

WEBER:

A practical consideration in the use of the transdermal preparation is choosing an appropriate part of the body on which it can be placed. It has been recommended that the patch be placed either on the anterior chest wall or on the upper outer part of the arm. Professor Rowland's data indicate that the medication diffuses satisfactorily through the skin at these sites. Should these parts of the body prove not to be practical or convenient for a particular patient, are there any reasonable alternatives?

ROWLAND:

It is generally accepted that the chest wall and the upper arm are the best places to apply the transdermal preparation, but there have not yet been sufficient good comparative studies to determine the feasibility of other sites. We did a study comparing the effects of the transdermal clonidine administered on the thigh. In that instance, the plasma concentrations of clonidine were significantly lower than those found during administration to the chest or arm. The clinical significance of this difference, specifically the possible change in blood pressure in hypertensive patients, has not yet been evaluated. I should like to see more investigations of this type carried out for two reasons. Firstly, I would like to compare the antihypertensive efficacy of transdermal clonidine systems applied to different parts of the body, and secondly, I would be very interested in learning whether the potential for skin reactions is the same on all parts of the body. Some of the earlier discussions during the symposium made it clear that there is much we do not yet know about what precipitates skin reactions during this type of treatment, and it might be useful to perform some further simple studies of the type I mentioned earlier.

CALNAN:

As a dermatologist, I support what Professor Rowland has suggested. Both the outer arm and the chest are areas that do seem susceptible to skin reactions. It would be interesting to see further studies where the thigh or other parts of the body are used as the sites of application for transdermal medication. For instance, the abdomen could be tested as a site for this form of treatment.

Author Index

Subject Index

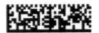